A STEREOTAXIC ATLAS OF THE BRAIN OF THE CEBUS MONKEY

(*CEBUS APELLA*)

SOHAN L. MANOCHA

TOTADA R. SHANTHA

GEOFFREY H. BOURNE

Yerkes Regional Primate Research Center, Emory University, Atlanta, Georgia, U.S.A.

OXFORD · AT THE CLARENDON PRESS
1968

Oxford University Press, Ely House, London W. I

GLASGOW NEW YORK TORONTO MELBOURNE WELLINGTON
CAPE TOWN SALISBURY IBADAN NAIROBI LUSAKA ADDIS ABABA
BOMBAY CALCUTTA MADRAS KARACHI LAHORE DACCA
KUALA LUMPUR HONG KONG TOKYO

Preface

THE primary objective of this stereotaxic atlas is to map out anatomically the various nuclei and fibre systems and to provide a detailed Horsley–Clarke co-ordinate system of the brain of the Cebus Monkey (*Cebus apella*). The Cebus Monkey is an alert, mechanically skilful, and intelligent animal. It is fairly resistant to common laboratory infections and can be purchased and maintained at a comparatively low cost. Its easy availability from South American countries makes it an animal of choice in many experiments as an alternative to the Squirrel and Rhesus Monkeys. The latter is becoming increasingly difficult and expensive to import from India. This base-line neuroanatomical study is expected to provide a useful tool for further neuroanatomical, neurophysiological, and related types of work. It should also be of value to students of neuroanatomy who are interested in learning about the various nuclei and fibre systems of a sub-human primate brain.

This work was supported by Grant FR-00165, Animal Resources Branch, National Institutes of Health, and NASA Grant 11-001-016. We are thankful to Dr. Adrian Perachio for his assistance in checking the stereotaxic levels and to Mrs. Astrid Jackson for help in preparation of the manuscript. Dr. T. R. Shanthaveerappa in previous publications is here referred to as Dr. T. R. Shantha.

SOHAN L. MANOCHA, Ph.D.

TOTADA R. SHANTHA,* M.D., Ph.D.

GEOFFREY H. BOURNE, Sc.D., D.Phil.

Yerkes Regional Primate Research Center
Emory University
Atlanta, Georgia 30322 U.S.A.

* T. R. SHANTHAVEERAPPA in previous publications.

Contents

1. Introduction

Cebus apella, commonly called the 'Brown' or 'Tufted' Capuchin Monkey, has been a primate of choice in many laboratories for various experimental purposes. Its easy availability from the South American continent makes it an ideal substitute for the Rhesus species, which is becoming increasingly difficult to obtain from eastern countries due to numerous transportation and import problems. The Squirrel Monkey, another New World primate, although easily available, is not as intelligent as the Capuchin Monkey, which is sometimes referred to as a 'mechanical genius'. Its low cost and reasonably high intellectual capacity and skill (Klüver 1935, 1937) make it all the more attractive for planning experiments requiring the use of large numbers of animals. Also, the Capuchin Monkey is fairly resistant to common infections and is easier to handle and less bulky than the Macaques, thereby posing fewer problems of caging, maintenance, and handling.

So far there has been no systematic study of the central nervous system (CNS) of this animal. A short report on the stereotaxic levels, with line drawings through the anterior part (from A19·0 to A2·0) of the Cebus brain, has been published by Eidelberg and Saldias (1960). This report, however, is lacking in anatomical details of the various diencephalic and brain-stem nuclei and of the various fibre systems. It is imperative, therefore, to have a detailed Horsley–Clarke co-ordinate type of atlas if this animal is to be used for neurophysiological, experimental, neuroanatomical, and related types of work. An attempt has been made in the present atlas to identify and label the various nuclei and fibre systems. It is believed that this stereotaxic study will serve as a useful base-line for different types of experiments on the CNS of this animal, and for comparison with other species.

Terminology used in this atlas is based on *Nomina Anatomica* as also used by Snider and Lee (1961), Emmers and Akert (1963), and Shantha *et al.* (1968).

2. Geographical distribution of *Cebus apella*

THIS species of Capuchin Monkey is widely distributed in Latin America. It is found in the southern part of Central America, north-western Colombia, Paraguay, and the extreme south-east of Brazil adjoining the Argentine territory of Misiones. It is also found in eastern Brazil around Pernambuco and extending northward beyond Miritiba (Hill 1960).

C. apella apella is concentrated in the Guianas and extends southward and eastward to Brazil. *C. a. margaritae* is found in Margarita Island and Venezuela. *C. a. fatuellus* is mainly concentrated in eastern Colombia and on the lower slopes of the Andes. *C. a. tocantinus* is found around the mouth of Rio Tocantins. *C. a. macrocephalus* is found mainly in the upper Amazon basin. *C. a. magnus* inhabits the western Colombian Andes, extending northward into southern Central America. *C. a. juruanus* is found on the banks of Rio Jurua. *C. a. maranonis* is distributed in Columbia and north-eastern Peru. *C. a. peruanus* is concentrated in eastern Peru and the extreme west of Brazil. *C. a. pallidus* is found in Bolivia in the Rio Beni and Rio Mamore drainage areas. *C. a. cay* is distributed between Rio Parana and Rio Paraguay. *C. a. libidinosus* is found in east central Brazil along the left bank of Rio São Francisco. *C. a. xanthosternos* is mainly concentrated between the east coast of Brazil and the right bank of Rio São Francisco. *C. a. robustus* is found mainly in eastern Brazil. *C. a. frontatus* is concentrated in Vieira, whereas *C. a. nigritus* is mainly found in eastern Brazil (Hill 1960).

2

3. Species characteristics

THE main species of Capuchin Monkeys are *Cebus apella*, *Cebus albifrons*, *Cebus capucinus*, *Cebus fatuellus*, *Cebus hypoleucus*, *Cebus griseus*, *Cebus nigrivittatus*, etc. The various Cebus species have been further grouped under Tufted (*C. apella*) and Untufted (*C. capucinus*, *C. albifrons*, *C. nigrivittatus*) Capuchins (Hershkovitz 1949, Hill 1960). A similar distinction between the Tufted and Untufted species of the Cebus group was earlier made by Tate (1939) on the basis of their being either 'Crested' or 'Uncrested'. The main differences, as described by Hershkovitz (1949), between the Tufted and Untufted groups are summarized below.

Tufted	*Untufted*
1. Temporal ridges more developed and convergent, uniting in old males to form a sagittal crest.	Temporal ridges weakly developed, never converging to form a sagittal crest.
2. Superciliary ridges weak.	Well defined, nearly horizontal superciliary ridges.
3. Brain case more vaulted, less dolichocephalic.	Brain case relatively low and dolichocephalic.
4. Ramus of the mandible in males comparatively high.	Ramus of the mandible in males comparatively low.
5. Vomer situated more anteriorly and not exposed behind the plane of the posterior border of the palate.	Vomer situated more posteriorly and always exposed behind the plane of the posterior border of the palate.
6. Frontal tufts usually present in both sexes and may have different shapes.	Frontal tufts normally absent in males and when present in females they are placed well forward in the form of a superciliary brush or frontal diadem.
7. Caps of crown always broad and never pointed or wedge-shaped in front.	Caps of crowns are either broad or narrow, and may also be rounded or pointed in front.
8. A dark preauricular band present on both sides of the face.	Dark preauricular band absent.
9. They are said to have 5 lumbar and 12-13 thoracic vertebrae.	They are believed to have 6 lumbar and 14-15 thoracic vertebrae.

Species characteristics

The species *Cebus apella* belonging to the Tufted group has been selected on the basis of its wider distribution and easy availability. It is believed that, in spite of the above-mentioned species-differences between the members of the Tufted and Untufted groups, the present neuroanatomical atlas can be used for all Capuchin Monkeys.

Cebus apella is distinct as a group, but a few workers (Hershkovitz 1949, Hill 1960) still recognize minor differences within this species and have further classified it into a number of subspecies (*Cebus apella apella, C. a. margaritae, C. a. fatuellus, C. a. tocantinus, C. a. macrocephalus, C. a. magnus, C. a. juruanus, C. a. maranonis, C. a. peruanus, C. a. pallidus, C. a. cay, C. a. libidinosus, C. a. xanthosternos, C. a. robustus, C. a. frontatus, C. a. nigritus*). This classification is based on local specializations in hair patterns (tracts of larger hairs), particularly on each side of the crown patch, as well as different geographical distribution in the South American continent. The identity of *Cebus apella* as a single composite unit as a member of the Tufted group is, therefore, undisputed.

4. External morphology of the brain

THE Capuchin Monkey brain is typical of a mammalian species and can be divided into frontal, parietal, temporal, and occipital lobes (Figs. 1 and 2). The fissura centralis on the lateral surface, dividing the frontal from the parietal lobe, is quite prominent. Anterior to the central sulcus (*slc*), the lateral and orbital surfaces of the frontal lobe show the sulcus precentralis superior (*pcs*) and precentralis inferior or arcuate (*pc*), sulcus rectus (*sr*), and sulcus orbitalis (*o*), as observed in the Macaque brain. The sulcus precentralis inferior presents a horizontal limb (*sph*) at its superior extremity and is located dorsal to the sulcus rectus. The sulcus subcentralis anterior, found in between the sulcus precentralis inferior and the lower end of the sulcus centralis, is an indistinct ill-defined sulcus compared to that of Rhesus (*Macaca mulatta*). The sulcus rectus (*sr*) is constantly found in the various animals used in the present study and is well marked. The area of the frontal lobe in between *slc*, *pcs*, and *pc* represents the gyrus precentralis (*gpc*). The *sr* located anterior to *pcs* and *pc* divides the frontal lobe into the upper and lower parts. The upper part contains both the gyri frontalis medialis (*gfm*) and frontalis superior (*gfs*), separated by an indistinct sulcus arising from *sr*. The lower part is the gyrus frontalis inferior (*gfi*).

The sulcus orbitalis (*o*) is represented as a tri-radiate or Y-shaped structure, with one limb comparatively ill-defined. The sulcus olfactorius, with its ill-defined segment, divides the orbital division of the frontal lobe into medially-placed gyrus rectus (*gr*) and laterally-placed gyrus orbitalis (*go*). As observed in other primates, this nerve divides posteriorly into medial and lateral striae. The latter disappears above the uncus, whereas the medial stria can be traced up to the gyrus subcallosus—a gyrus which is formed below the rostrum of the corpus callosum. The medial and lateral striae, along with the diagonal band of Broca (which is the posterior boundary), form the anterior perforated substance.

The sulcus centralis (*slc*), which divides the frontal from the parietal lobe, is deep and well marked on the lateral surface and is very superficial on the medial surface. The parietal surface presents a well-defined sulcus intraparietalis (*sip*), which joins at its convexity with the lower end of the sulcus parieto-occipitalis (*poc*). This sulcus continues for a short distance into the occipital area as ramus occipitalis or par-occipitalis (*par*). The sulcus par-occipitalis continues into sulcus lunatus (*l*) to form a prominent concavo-convex sulcus on the occipital lobe. The sulcus lunatus (*l*) gives a short anterior branch called sulcus prelunatus (*pl*) at its lower part. Connolly (1950) has, however, shown the sulcus lunatus as a separate sulcus not joining the par-occipitalis in the

Cebus brain (Connolly, Fig. 16, p. 21). This observation was also made in some brains used in the present study.

The sulcus occipitalis inferior (*oc*) runs close to the ventral border below the sulcus lunatus and gives off a short segment at its anterior end. The lateral surface of the occipital lobe extends ventral to the sulcus occipitalis inferior and anterior to the sulcus lunatus. This striate area is smooth and unbroken by any fissurations.

The fissura Sylvii (*fs*) joins the parallel sulcus or the sulcus temporalis superior (*sts*) at the posterior end. The *sts* extends upward towards the apex of the sulcus intraparietalis (*sip*). At its anterior end *fs* and *sts* are separated by the grey matter of the gyrus temporalis superior (*gts*). The sulcus temporalis medianus (*tm*) is found at the anterior or temporal pole of the temporal lobe and is represented by a small, approximately 12-mm long, sulcus. The anterior part is deeper than the posterior part.

Posterior to the fissura centralis lies the gyrus postcentralis (*gyp*), which is the most anterior part of the parietal lobe. The insula is hidden under the fissura Sylvii (*fs*). The *fs*, *sts*, and *tm* divide the temporal lobe into gyrus temporalis superior (*gts*), gyrus temporalis medius (*gtm*), and gyrus temporalis inferior (*gti*). Because of the shortness of the *tm*, the posterior part of the inferior temporal lobe merges with the middle temporal lobe. The region between the sulcus intraparietalis (*sip*) and the confluence of *fs* and *ts* is termed the gyrus angularis (*ga*). The dorsal aspect of the parietal lobe, which is found immediately in front of the *poc* and the rostral limb of *sip*, has been named the gyrus parietalis anterior (*gpa*).

On the medial surface (Fig. 2), the sulcus calloso-marginalis (*scm*) starts from a point above and anterior to the genu of the corpus callosum (*cc*), and extends posteriorly to a point just above the splenium. The posterior one-third of the sulcus runs upwards and backwards towards the medial border. Ventral to the *scm* is located the gyrus callosus marginalis (*gcm*). Dorsal to the *scm* the extension of the motor area as well as the gyrus frontalis superior (*gfs*) are located. Between the ventral and anterior part of corpus callosum bounded by the anterior segment of the *scm* and *rs*, lies the gyrus callosus (*gyc*).

The sulcus rostralis (*rs*) is found anterior to the genu of the corpus callosum and runs parallel to the medial orbital margin, with its convexity pointing upwards. The sulcus subparietalis (*ssp*) is found posterior to the *scm* and runs almost parallel to its posterior segment. At about its middle a small ramus is given off.

The internal part of the sulcus parieto-occipitalis (*spo*) is quite prominent in the

Cebus and runs downwards and backwards with its concavity directed upwards. At its lower end it meets the posterior end of the sulcus paracalcarinus (*pca*). Connolly (1950) has, however, shown that in the Cebus brain the *spo* does not join the *pca* at its lower end. Instead, the *pca* is shown as an independent semicircular sulcus (Connolly, Fig. 17, p. 21). The sulcus paracalcarinus is also known as the ventral element of the parieto-occipital fissure.

The sulcus retrocalcarinus (*rc*) is well developed in Cebus and is represented by an almost straight groove that terminates caudally with a vertically running sulcus forming a letter 'T'. The sulcus calcarinus lateralis (*scl*) is found at the occipital pole of the occipital lobe and extends for a short distance both on the medial and supero-lateral surfaces of the occipital lobe. This sulcus is very superficial compared to the sulcus retrocalcarinus (*rc*). The posterior segment of the sulcus occipitalis inferior (*oci*) also extends to the medial surface of the occipital lobe at its lower part, below the sulcus calcarinus lateralis (*scl*). The *spo* and the *rc* with its rostral limb form the boundary of the cuneus area, whereas the *rc* along with its caudal limb encloses the gyrus lingualis (*gyl*). The boundary between the gyrus lingualis and gyrus hippocampus is confluent and is hard to differentiate because of the absence of any surface markings. The gyrus hippocampus is bounded anteriorly and laterally by the fissura rhinalis. The area between the fissura collateralis and *oci* has been said to represent an area which is homologous to the gyrus fusiformis of man (Hines 1933).

On the inferior surface of the brain the sulcus occipito-temporalis is well marked. Posteriorly it joins the sulcus retrocalcarinus almost at the middle of the latter.

A general comparison of the Cebus (Platyrrhine) brain with that of Macaca (Catarrhine) reveals that there is a considerable difference in the degree of fissuration. The Macaque brain on the average is better fissurated than the Cebus even when comparing brains of the same size in both the species. The post-central superior sulcus is well marked in the Macaques but is rarely present in the Cebus. Even when present, this sulcus is represented by a mere dimple. The consistent presence of this sulcus in the Macaque clearly indicates further cortical differentiation than in the Cebus. The intraparietal sulcus is larger and more sinuous in the Macaque, compared to a short and less sinuous one in the Cebus. The frontal sulci are also less developed in the Cebus than in the Macaque. The vertical part of the sulcus precentralis inferior or arcuate is farther away from the central sulcus in the Cebus than in the Macaque brain, where it shows a tendency to closer proximity to the central sulcus.

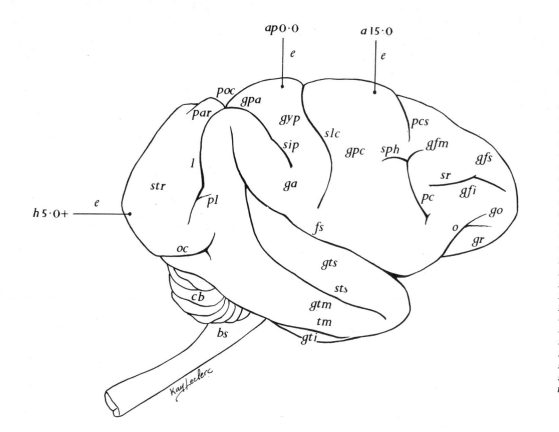

bs	Brain stem
cb	Cerebellum
e	Electrode
fs	Fissura Sylvii
ga	Gyrus angularis
gfi	Gyrus frontalis inferior
gfm	Gyrus frontalis medialis
gfs	Gyrus frontalis superior
go	Gyrus orbitalis
gpa	Gyrus parietalis anterior
gpc	Gyrus precentralis
gr	Gyrus rectus
gti	Gyrus temporalis inferior
gtm	Gyrus temporalis medius
gts	Gyrus temporalis superior
gyp	Gyrus postcentralis
l	Sulcus lunatus
o	Sulcus orbitalis
oc	Sulcus occipitalis inferior
par	Ramus occipitalis
pc	Sulcus precentralis inferior
pcs	Sulcus precentralis superior
pl	Sulcus prelunatus
poc	Fissura and sulcus parieto-occipitalis
sip	Sulcus intraparietalis
slc	Sulcus centralis
sph	Sulcus precentralis inferior—horizontal part
sr	Sulcus rectus
str	Striate area
sts	Sulcus temporalis superior
tm	Sulcus temporalis medianus

FIG. 1. Lateral view of brain of Cebus monkey

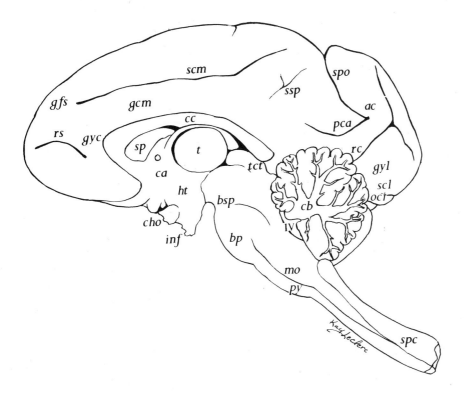

ac	Area cuneus
bp	Brachium pontis
bsp	Basis pedunculi cerebri
ca	Commissura anterior
cb	Cerebellum
cc	Corpus callosum
cho	Chiasma nervorum opticorum
gcm	Gyrus callosus marginalis
gfs	Gyrus frontalis superior
gyc	Gyrus callosus
gyl	Gyrus lingualis
ht	Area hypothalamicus
inf	Infundibulum
mo	Medulla oblongata
oci	Sulcus occipitalis inferior
pca	Sulcus paracalcarinus
py	Pyramid
rc	Sulcus retrocalcarinus
rs	Sulcus rostralis
scl	Sulcus calcarinus lateralis
scm	Sulcus calloso-marginalis
sp	Septum pellucidum
spc	Spinal cord
spo	Sulcus parieto-occipitalis
ssp	Sulcus subparietalis
t	Thalamus
tct	Tectum
IV	Ventriculus quartus

FIG. 2. Mid-sagittal section of brain of Cebus Monkey

5. Materials and methods

A. Material

FIVE animals of both sexes, weighing from 2·0 to 2·9 kg and with healthy coats, were selected. Before being killed, the animals were tested for various parasitic infestations and other infections. They were anaesthetized with sodium pentobarbital, given intraperitoneally. The head of the anaesthetized animal was perfused with normal saline, first through cannulae inserted in the common carotid artery, and then in the jugular vein. This process was repeated on the opposite side. The saline perfusion was continued until the extruding fluid became colourless, and was then followed by perfusion with 10 per cent formalin (unbuffered). The perfusion was continued overnight, with the head submerged in 10 per cent formalin.

The head was cut off the animal's body and the skull cap was removed with an electric saw. The dura mater was slit open at a number of places to allow direct contact with the fixative. The heads were then stored in freshly prepared 10 per cent formalin for a couple of weeks until they were ready to be used. The brains were removed, after inserting the electrodes at appropriate places as described below. The brain weight ranged from 60 to 66 g. The length of the brains ranged from 60·5 to 62·0 mm and the breadth from 50 to 52 mm.

B. Stereotaxic technique

The David Kopf stereotaxic instrument was used. As usual, the head was fixed firmly in the instrument before reference electrodes were introduced. The lower jaw was purposely kept wide open, by inserting a paper ball into it when the animal was killed, to facilitate the positioning of the mouth bar of the stereotaxic instrument.

The antero-posterior zero plane (APO·O) is represented by a straight line passing through the width of the brain through the centre of the external auditory meati. The coronal sections represented in this atlas anterior to this APO·O plane are marked A and the posterior P. Each number indicates the distance in millimetres anterior and posterior to this plane.

In addition to the pair of electrodes inserted vertically (coronal) at APO·O, a number of reference electrodes on both sides of the left and right planes were also implanted at different distances anterior and posterior to APO·O. These reference electrodes served as additional guide lines to determine the various stereotaxic levels during the sectioning process.

Horizontal electrodes were also introduced at a level 15 mm above the Frankfurt plane. The Frankfurt plane, or the basi-horizontal plane, is the plane represented by a line passing through the centre of the external auditory meati and the lower margin of the orbital opening. The horizontal 0 plane (HO·0) is the straight line that passes through the cranium 10 mm above, and parallel to, the Frankfurt plane. This level is also known as the Horsley–Clarke plane. The measurements above this HO·0 plane have been marked as + (plus) and the levels below this plane as − (minus).

The left–right 0 plane (LRO·0) is a plane passing through the sagittal plane of the brain, dividing it into symmetrical right and left halves. Most of the photographs used in this atlas show the left half of the brain. Each division of the scale indicated on the plates represents magnification of 1 mm distance.

The path of the horizontal electrode was marked by injecting a 10 per cent solution of activated charcoal in propylene glycol. The deposited carbon particles have proved in this study to be an ideal indicator of the electrode track. This material was injected drop by drop while the already-introduced hollow electrode needles were being withdrawn. In the case of vertical electrodes implanted at A22·0 and P12·0, the inserted needles were clothed with polyethylene tubing of appropriate size. While the steel needles were being withdrawn, the plastic tubes were left behind. These tubes *in situ* served as guide lines for cutting the anterior and posterior ends of the brain.

C. Sectioning of the brain

After the electrodes were implanted as described above, the brain was removed from the skull cavity with minimum injury to the surface of the brain. The meninges and the blood-vessels were meticulously cleaned away from the brain with the help of a fine forceps. The brain was sliced vertically along the plastic tubes previously left in the brain at the time of fixing the electrodes. This procedure facilitated slicing the brain vertically, which in turn helped in getting the frontal section parallel to the vertically implanted electrodes. The brain was cut anteriorly at A22·0 and posteriorly at P12·0. Two to three blocks were cut at varying levels in different brains in order to prepare a complete series of sections through the entire length of the brain. These blocks were further fixed in 10 per cent formalin for at least 48 h. The desired block was then put in a mixture of 20 cm³ absolute alcohol and 80 cm³ 10 per cent formalin for 24 h at 40° C, as described by Marshall (1940). Without any washing the block was frozen in dry ice and mounted on the cryostat chuck. Series of 40-μm-thick sections were cut out of similarly processed blocks of tissue in a cryostat at -20 to $-25°$ C. The sections were mounted on pre-cleaned albumin-coated pre-cooled slides. The sections were floated in 10 per cent formalin to remove the trapped air bubbles and to stretch out any wrinkles in the sections. The excess formalin was blotted out.

The sections were serially numbered, and an attempt was made to use all the sections except those badly torn in the process of cutting. Sections were dried overnight at $37°$ C before staining.

D. Staining of the sections

The mounted sections were stained both for nerve-fibre systems (Weil method) and for cellular systems (Nissl method). The following procedures were employed.

1. *Weil method*

Staining solution:

95 per cent ethanol solution of 10 per cent haematoxylin diluted to 1 per cent solution with distilled water + equal volume of differentiating solution A.

Differentiating solutions:

A = 4 per cent ferric ammonium sulphate.

B = equal parts of 20 per cent tetrasodium borate, 25 per cent potassium ferri-cyanide, and distilled water.

Steps:

(1) Slides placed in 95 per cent alcohol for from 2 h to overnight;

(2) hydrated in 70–30 per cent alcohol–tap-water for 5–10 min each;

(3) placed in staining solution at 45–$50°$ C for 75–90 min;

(4) washed in 3 changes of tap-water;

(5) differentiated in solution A for 5–20 min (till cellular areas became light grey);

(6) washed in running tap-water;

(7) differentiated in solution B for 2–10 min;

(8) washed in running tap-water;

(9) dehydrated 30–70–95 per cent alcohol for 5–10 min each;

(10) absolute alcohol for 5–10 min, 2 changes;

(11) cleared in xylene;

(12) mounted in DPX or Canada balsam.

2. *Nissl method*

Staining solution:

1 per cent cresyl violet solution or the following mixture:

$$cresyl\ violet = 1\ g,$$
$$distilled\ water = 1000\ cm^3,$$
$$glacial\ acetic\ acid = 3.1\ cm^3,$$
$$sodium\ acetate = 0.205\ g.$$

Steps:

(1) Sections hydrated in 95–70–35 per cent alcohol–distilled water for 5–10 min each;

(2) stained for 3–6 min at room temperature and rinsed in 70 per cent alcohol for 2–5 min;

(3) differentiated in 95 per cent ethanol till the required contrast was obtained;

(4) dehydrated in 2 changes of ethyl alcohol for 5–10 min;

(5) cleared in xylene;

(6) mounted in DPX or Canada balsam.

When 1 per cent cresyl violet solution was used 20–30 drops of glacial acetic acid were added to the 1000 cm^3 of 95 per cent alcohol while differentiating.

Occasionally, due to unknown reasons, the Nissl staining faded and diffused into the surrounding unstained areas of the section within a week after mounting. Those slides were reprocessed and stained again with Nissl stain.

E. Photography

The sections were photographed by our enlarger method described earlier (Shantha-veerappa *et al.* 1965). The mounted slides were inserted in the negative carrier plate and mounted into the photographic enlarger. A 4 × 5-in. film was exposed in the manner of printing paper for half a second. The exposed films were processed and the prints were made from these negatives. All the figures of the original stained-brain preparations given in this atlas are evenly magnified six and two-thirds times. The Nissl- and Weil-stained preparations belonging to the same stereotaxic level have been arranged on opposite pages. The plates are arranged in sequence from A19·5 to P9·0.

Bibliography

ANDY, O. J., and STEPHAN, H. (1961). Septal nuclei in the Soricidae (insectivors). Cyto-architectonic study. *J. comp. Neurol.* **117**, 251-74.

ANGEVINE, J. B., Jr., MANCALL, E. L., and YAKOVLEV, P. I. (1961). *The human cerebellum. An atlas of gross topography in serial sections.* Little, Brown & Co., Boston.

ATLAS, D. H., and INGRAM, W. R. (1937). Topography of the brain stem of the rhesus monkey with special reference to the diencephalon. *J. comp. Neurol.* **66**, 263-99.

BERKE, J. J. (1960). The claustrum, the external capsule and the extreme capsule of *Macaca mulatta.* Ibid. **115**, 297-321.

BONIN, G. VON (1938). The cerebral cortex of the cebus monkey. Ibid. **69**, 181-227.

BRUCE, A. (1901). *A topographical atlas of the spinal cord.* William & Norgate, Oxford.

CASTELLANOS, J. J. (1949*a*). Thalamus of the cat in Horsley–Clarke coordinates. *J. comp. Neurol.* **91**, 307-39.

——— (1949*b*). The amygdaloid complex in monkey studied by reconstitutional methods. Ibid. 506-26.

CHIRO, G. DI (1961). *An atlas of detailed normal pneumoencephalographic anatomy.* Thomas, Springfield, Illinois.

CLARK, W. E. LEGROS (1932). The structure and connections of the thalamus. *Brain* **55**, 406-70.

CLARKE, R. H. (1920). Investigation of the central nervous system. Methods and instruments. *Johns Hopkins Hospital Reports*, Special Volume, Part 1, pp. 1-160.

CONNOLLY, C. J. (1950). *External morphology of the primate brain.* Thomas, Springfield, Illinois.

DEKABAN, A. (1953). Human thalamus. An anatomical, developmental and pathological study. I. Division of the human adult thalamus into nuclei by the use of cyto-myelo-architectonic methods. *J. comp. Neurol.* **99**, 639-83.

DELMAS, A., and PERTUISET, B. (1959). *Cranio-cerebral topometry in man.* Masson, Paris; Thomas, Springfield, Illinois.

DELUCCHI, M. R., DENNIS, B. V., and ADEY, W. R. (1965). A stereotaxic atlas of the chimpanzee brain (*Pan satyrus*). University of California Press, Los Angeles.

DUMITRESCU, H. (1959). *Atlas citoarchitectonic al creierului de Cobai.* Editura Academiei Republicii Populare Romine.

EIDELBERG, E., and SALDIAS, C. A. (1960). Stereotaxic atlas for Cebus Monkeys. *J. comp. Neurol.* **115**, 103-24.

EMMERS, R., and AKERT, K. (1963). *A stereotaxic atlas of the brain of Squirrel Monkey.* The University of Wisconsin Press, Madison.

FRONTERA, J. G. (1958). Evaluation of the immediate effects of some fixatives upon the measurements of the brains of macaques. *J. comp. Neurol.* **109**, 417-38.

GEIST, F. D. (1930). The brain of the Rhesus Monkey. Ibid. **50**, 333-75.

GERGEN, J. A., and MACLEAN, P. D. (1962). A stereotaxic atlas of the Squirrel Monkey brain. *U.S. Public Health Service Publication*, No. 933.

HERSHKOVITZ, P. (1949). Mammals of northern Columbia. Preliminary report No. 4: Monkeys (primates) with taxonomic revisions of some forms. *Proc. U.S. natn. Mus.* **98,** 323–427.

HILL, W. C. O. (1960). *Primates, comparative anatomy and taxonomy. IV. Cebidae.* Part A. University Press, Edinburgh.

HINES, M. (1933). The external morphology of the brain and the spinal cord. Hartman and Strauss's *Anatomy of the rhesus monkey*, pp. 275–89. William & Wilkins, Baltimore.

INGRAM, W. R. (1940). Nuclear organization and chief connections of the primate hypothalamus. Fulton, Ranson, and Frantz's *The hypothalamus and central levels of autonomic function*, pp. 195–244. William & Wilkins, Baltimore.

JASPER, H. H., and AJMONE-MARSAN, C. (1956). *A stereotaxic atlas of the diencephalon of the cat.* National Research Council of Canada, Ottawa.

KLÜVER, H. (1935). *Behavior mechanisms in monkeys.* University of Chicago Press.

—— (1937). Reexamination of implement-using behavior in a Cebus Monkey. *Acta psychol.* **2,** 347–97.

KÖNIG, J. F. R., and KLIPPEL, R. A. (1963). *The rat brain. Stereotaxic atlas of the forebrain and lower parts of the brain stem.* William & Wilkins, Baltimore.

KRIEG, W. J. S. (1948). A reconstruction of the diencephalic nuclei of *Macaca rhesus.* *J. comp. Neurol.* **88,** 1–52.

MARSHALL, W. H. (1940). An application of the frozen sectioning technique for cutting serial sections through the brain. *Stain Technol.* **15,** 133–8.

McCORMICK, J. B., and BLATT, M. B. (1961). *Atlas and demonstration technique of the central nervous system.* Thomas, Springfield, Illinois.

MEESEN, H., and OLSZEWSKI, J. (1949). *Cytoarchitectonic atlas of rhombencephalon of the rabbit.* Karger, Basle and New York.

MONNIER, M. (1949). *A short atlas of the brain stem of the cat and Rhesus Monkey for experimental research.* Springer-Verlag, Vienna.

—— and GANGLOFF, H. (1961). *Atlas for stereotaxic brain research on the conscious rabbit.* Elsevier; Amsterdam, London, and New York.

NOBACK, C. R. (1959). Brain of a gorilla. II. Brain stem nuclei. *J. comp. Neurol.* **111,** 345–86.

—— and GANDAL, C. (1960). The brain stem nuclei of the *Platypus-Ornithorhynchus anatinus. Anat. Rec.* **136,** 253.

OLSZEWSKI, J. (1952). *The thalamus of the* Macaca mulatta. Karger, Basle and New York.

—— and BAXTER, D. (1954). *Cytoarchitecture of the human brain stem.* Karger, Basle and New York.

PERACHIO, A. (1966). Sleep mechanisms in the primate brain. Ph.D. Dissertation, University of Rochester.

RILEY, H. L. (1960). *An atlas of the basal ganglia, brain stem and spinal cord.* Hafner, New York.

SCHALTENBRAND, G., and BAILEY, P. (1959). *Introduction to the stereotaxic operation and an atlas of the human brain.* Thieme, Stuttgart.

SHANTHAVEERAPPA, T. R., MANOCHA, S. L., and BOURNE, G. H. (1965). Macrophotography of thick sections and gels with a regular photographic enlarger. *Stain Technol.* **41,** 309.

SHANTHA, T. R., MANOCHA, S. L., and BOURNE, G. H. (1968). *A stereotaxic atlas of the Java Monkey brain* (Macaca irus). Karger, Basle and New York.

SHANZER, S., and WAGMAN, I. H. (1960). A method for the determination of the horizontal plane in *M. mulatta. Electroenceph. clin. Neurophysiol.* **12,** 214-16.

SHEPS, J. G. (1945). The nuclear configuration and cortical connections of the human thalamus. *J. comp. Neurol.* **83,** 1-56.

SINGER, M. (1962). *The brain of the dog in section.* Saunders, Philadelphia and London.

—— and YAKOVLEV, P. I. (1964). *The human brain in sagittal section.* Thomas, Springfield, Illinois.

SNIDER, R. S., and LEE, J. C. (1961). *A stereotaxic atlas of the monkey brain* (Macaca mulatta). University of Chicago Press.

—— and NIEMER, W. T. (1961). *A stereotaxic atlas of the cat brain.* University of Chicago Press.

STEPHAN, H., and ANDY, O. J. (1964). Cytoarchitectonics of the septal nuclei in Old World monkeys (Cercopithecus and Colobus). *J. Hirnforsch.* **7,** 1-8.

TABER, E., BRODAL, A., and WALBERG, F. (1960). The raphe nuclei of the brain stem in the cat. I. Normal topography and cyto-architecture and general discussion. *J. comp. Neurol.* **114,** 161.

TATE, G. H. H. (1939). The mammals of the Guiana region. *Bull. Am. Mus. nat. Hist.* **76,** 151-229.

WEIL, A. A. (1928). A rapid method for staining myelin sheaths. *Archs. Neurol. Psychiat., Chicago,* **20,** 392-3.

WINCKLER, C., and POTTER, A. (1914). *Anatomical guide to experimental researches on the cat's brain.* Versluys, Amsterdam.

Bibliography

16

PHOTOGRAPHS OF CORONAL BRAIN SECTIONS
IN STEREOTAXIC CO-ORDINATES

aaa	Area anterior amygdalae
aca	Area claustralis amygdalae
ba	Nucleus basalis amygdalae
baa	Nucleus basalis accessorius amygdalae
cag	Nucleus corticalis amygdalae
cc	Corpus callosum
cd	Nucleus caudatus
cea	Nucleus centralis amygdalae
cho	Chiasma nervorum opticorum
cis	Cortex insularis
cl	Claustrum
ctp	Cortex temporalis
ds	Nucleus dorsalis septi
e	Electrode track
gu	Gyrus uncinatus
ic	Insula Callejae
la	Nucleus lateralis amygdalae
ls	Nucleus lateralis septi
ma	Nucleus medialis amygdalae
ms	Nucleus medialis septi
nfdb	Nucleus fasciculi diagonalis Broca
put	Putamen
si	Substantia innominata
spa	Substantia perforata anterior
tof	Tuberculum olfactorium

A 19·5 W

ao	Area olfactoria
ase	Area septalis
cam	Corpus amygdalae
cc	Corpus callosum
cd	Nucleus caudatus
ce	Capsula externa
cet	Capsula extrema
cho	Chiasma nervorum opticorum
ci	Capsula interna
cor	Corona radiata
e	Electrode track
fdb	Fasciculus diagonalis Broca
fl	Fissura longitudinalis cerebri
fu	Fasciculus uncinatus
put	Putamen
sol	Stria olfactoria lateralis
som	Stria olfactoria medialis
II	Ventriculus lateralis

19

A 17·0 C

aaa   Area anterior amygdalae
ast   Nucleus accumbens septi
bal   Nucleus basalis accessorius lateralis amygdalae
bam   Nucleus basalis accessorius medialis amygdalae
bla   Nucleus basalis lateralis amygdalae
bm   Nucleus basalis (Meynert)
bma   Nucleus basalis medialis amygdalae
cag   Nucleus corticalis amygdalae
cc   Corpus callosum
cca   Cortex cingularis anterior
cd   Nucleus caudatus
cea   Nucleus centralis amygdalae
cho   Chiasma nervorum opticorum
cis   Cortex insularis
cl   Claustrum
ctp   Cortex temporalis
ds   Nucleus dorsalis septi
e   Electrode track
gp   Globus pallidus
gu   Gyrus uncinatus
la   Nucleus lateralis amygdalae
ls   Nucleus lateralis septi
ma   Nucleus medialis amygdalae
ms   Nucleus medialis septi
nca   Nucleus commissurae anterioris
nfdb   Nucleus fasciculi diagonalis Broca
pm   Nucleus praeopticus medianus
put   Putamen
si   Substantia innominata
tof   Tuberculum olfactorium

20

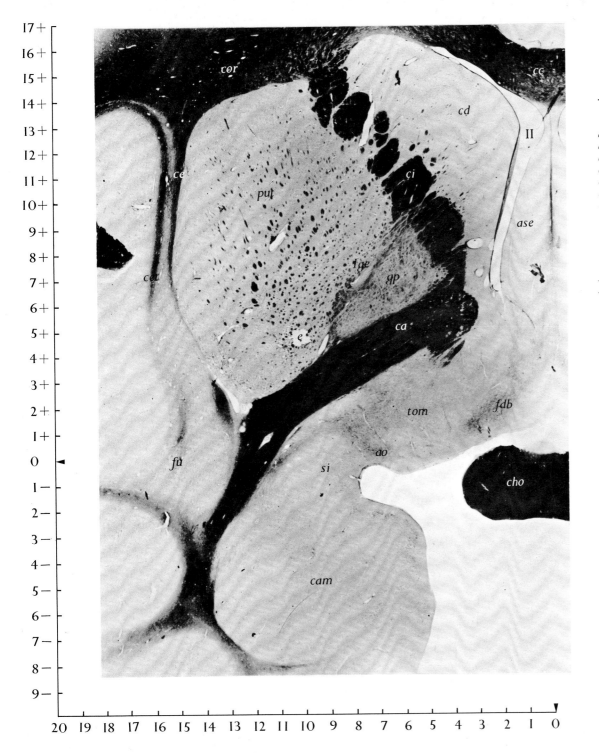

A 17·0 W

ao	Area olfactoria
ase	Area septalis
ca	Commissura anterior
cam	Corpus amygdalae
cc	Corpus callosum
cd	Nucleus caudatus
ce	Capsula externa
cet	Capsula extrema
cho	Chiasma nervorum opticorum
ci	Capsula interna
cor	Corona radiata
e	Electrode track
fdb	Fasciculus diagonalis Broca
fu	Fasciculus uncinatus
gp	Globus pallidus
lge	Globus pallidus, lamina medullaris externa
put	Putamen
si	Substantia innominata
tom	Tractus olfactomesencephalicus
II	Ventriculus lateralis

21

A 16·5 C

aaa	Area anterior amygdalae
apl	Area praeoptica lateralis
apm	Area praeoptica medialis
ast	Nucleus accumbens septi
baa	Nucleus basalis accessorius amygdalae
bla	Nucleus basalis lateralis amygdalae
bm	Nucleus basalis (Meynert)
bma	Nucleus basalis medialis amygdalae
cag	Nucleus corticalis amygdalae
cc	Corpus callosum
cd	Nucleus caudatus
cea	Nucleus centralis amygdalae
cho	Chiasma nervorum opticorum
cis	Cortex insularis
cl	Claustrum
ctp	Cortex temporalis
ds	Nucleus dorsalis septi
e	Electrode track
gp	Globus pallidus
gu	Gyrus uncinatus
la	Nucleus lateralis amygdalae
ls	Nucleus lateralis septi
ma	Nucleus medialis amygdalae
ms	Nucleus medialis septi
nca	Nucleus commissurae anterioris
nfdb	Nucleus fasciculi diagonalis Broca
pm	Nucleus praeopticus medianus
put	Putamen
si	Substantia innominata
tof	Tuberculum olfactorium

22

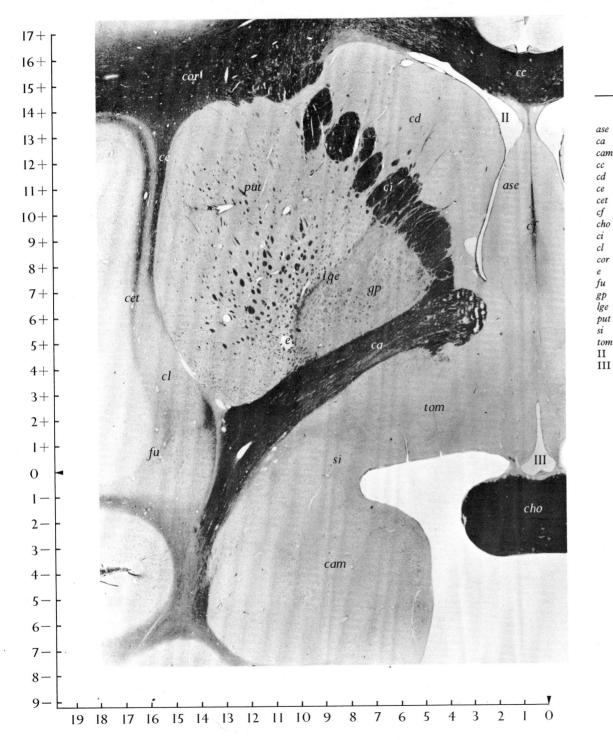

ase   Area septalis
ca   Commissura anterior
cam   Corpus amygdalae
cc   Corpus callosum
cd   Nucleus caudatus
ce   Capsula externa
cet   Capsula extrema
cf   Columna fornicis
cho   Chiasma nervorum opticorum
ci   Capsula interna
cl   Claustrum
cor   Corona radiata
e   Electrode track
fu   Fasciculus uncinatus
gp   Globus pallidus
lge   Globus pallidus, lamina medullaris externa
put   Putamen
si   Substantia innominata
tom   Tractus olfactomesencephalicus
II   Ventriculus lateralis
III   Ventriculus tertius

A 15·5 C

aaa   Area anterior amygdalae
ah   Nucleus anterior hypothalami
alh   Area lateralis hypothalami
amh   Area medialis hypothalami
baa   Nucleus basalis accessorius amygdalae
bla   Nucleus basalis lateralis amygdalae
bm   Nucleus basalis (Meynert)
bma   Nucleus basalis medialis amygdalae
cag   Nucleus corticalis amygdalae
cc   Corpus callosum
cd   Nucleus caudatus
cea   Nucleus centralis amygdalae
cho   Chiasma nervorum opticorum
cis   Cortex insularis
cl   Claustrum
cpf   Cortex piriformis
ctp   Cortex temporalis
ds   Nucleus dorsalis septi
e   Electrode track
gp   Globus pallidus
la   Nucleus lateralis amygdalae
ls   Nucleus lateralis septi
ma   Nucleus medialis amygdalae
ms   Nucleus medialis septi
nca   Nucleus commissurae anterioris
nfdb   Nucleus fasciculi diagonalis Broca
nst   Nucleus striae terminalis
pm   Nucleus praeopticus medianus
put   Putamen
sh   Nucleus suprachiasmaticus hypothalami
si   Substantia innominata
soh   Nucleus supraopticus hypothalami

24

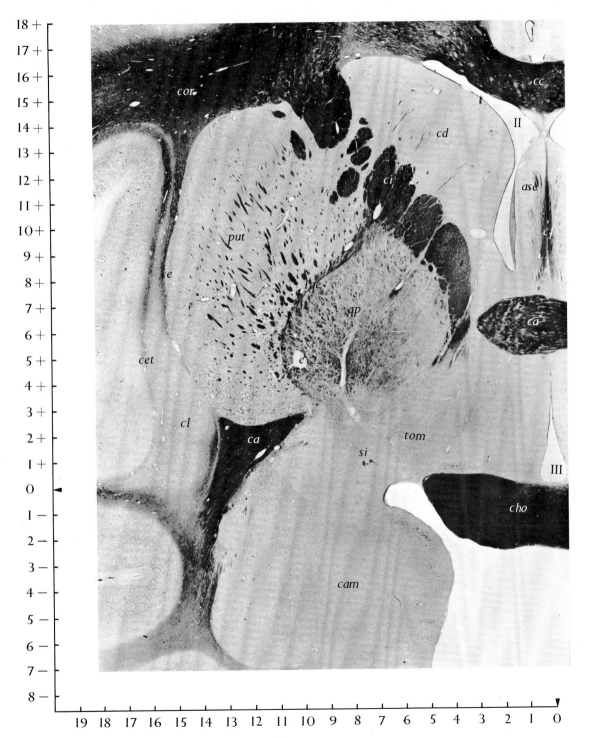

ase	Area septalis
ca	Commissura anterior
cam	Corpus amygdalae
cc	Corpus callosum
cd	Nucleus caudatus
ce	Capsula externa
cet	Capsula extrema
cf	Columna fornicis
cho	Chiasma nervorum opticorum
ci	Capsula interna
cl	Claustrum
cor	Corona radiata
e	Electrode track
gp	Globus pallidus
lge	Globus pallidus, lamina medullaris externa
put	Putamen
si	Substantia innominata
tom	Tractus olfactomesencephalicus
II	Ventriculus lateralis
III	Ventriculus tertius

A 14·5 C

adh   Area dorsalis hypothalami
alh   Area lateralis hypothalami
amh   Area medialis hypothalami
bal   Nucleus basalis accessorius lateralis amygdalae
bam   Nucleus basalis accessorius medialis amygdalae
bla   Nucleus basalis lateralis amygdalae
bm   Nucleus basalis (Meynert)
bma   Nucleus basalis medialis amygdalae
cag   Nucleus corticalis amygdalae
cc   Corpus callosum
cca   Cortex cingularis anterior
cd   Nucleus caudatus
cea   Nucleus centralis amygdalae
cis   Cortex insularis
cl   Claustrum
cpf   Cortex piriformis
ctp   Cortex temporalis
e   Electrode track
f   Fornix
gp   Globus pallidus
ica   Nucleus intercalatus amygdalae
la   Nucleus lateralis amygdalae
ma   Nucleus medialis amygdalae
nst   Nucleus striae terminalis
ph   Nucleus paraventricularis hypothalami
put   Putamen
sfo   Organum subfornicale
soh   Nucleus supraopticus hypothalami

26

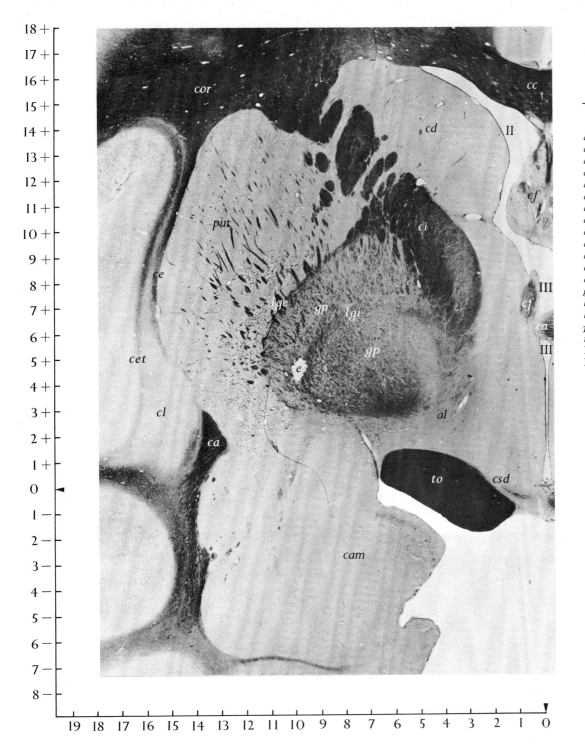

al   Ansa lenticularis
ca   Commissura anterior
cam   Corpus amygdalae
cc   Corpus callosum
cd   Nucleus caudatus
ce   Capsula externa
cet   Capsula extrema
cf   Columna fornicis
ci   Capsula interna
cl   Claustrum
cor   Corona radiata
csd   Commissura supraoptica dorsalis
e   Electrode track
gp   Globus pallidus
lge   Globus pallidus, lamina medullaris externa
lgi   Globus pallidus, lamina medullaris interna
put   Putamen
to   Tractus opticus
II   Ventriculus lateralis
III   Ventriculus tertius

adh	Area dorsalis hypothalami
alh	Area lateralis hypothalami
amh	Area medialis hypothalami
ba	Nucleus basalis amygdalae
baa	Nucleus basalis accessorius amygdalae
bm	Nucleus basalis (Meynert)
cag	Nucleus corticalis amygdalae
cc	Corpus callosum
cca	Cortex cingularis anterior
cd	Nucleus caudatus
cis	Cortex insularis
cl	Claustrum
cpf	Cortex piriformis
ctp	Cortex temporalis
e	Electrode track
em	Eminentia medialis
f	Fornix
gp	Globus pallidus
ica	Nucleus intercalatus amygdalae
ih	Nucleus infundibularis hypothalami
la	Nucleus lateralis amygdalae
ma	Nucleus medialis amygdalae
nst	Nucleus striae terminalis
ph	Nucleus paraventricularis hypothalami
put	Putamen
soh	Nucleus supraopticus hypothalami
trs	Nucleus triangularis septi

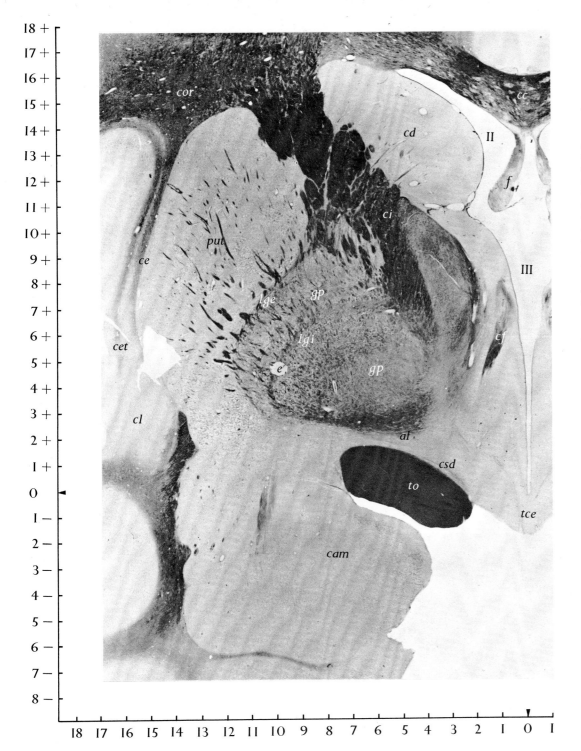

A 14·0 W

al Ansa lenticularis
cam Corpus amygdalae
cc Corpus callosum
cd Nucleus caudatus
ce Capsula externa
cet Capsula extrema
cf Columna fornicis
ci Capsula interna
cl Claustrum
cor Corona radiata
csd Commissura supraoptica dorsalis
e Electrode track
f Fornix
gp Globus pallidus
lge Globus pallidus, lamina medullaris externa
lgi Globus pallidus, lamina medullaris interna
put Putamen
tce Tuber cinereum
to Tractus opticus
II Ventriculus lateralis
III Ventriculus tertius

29

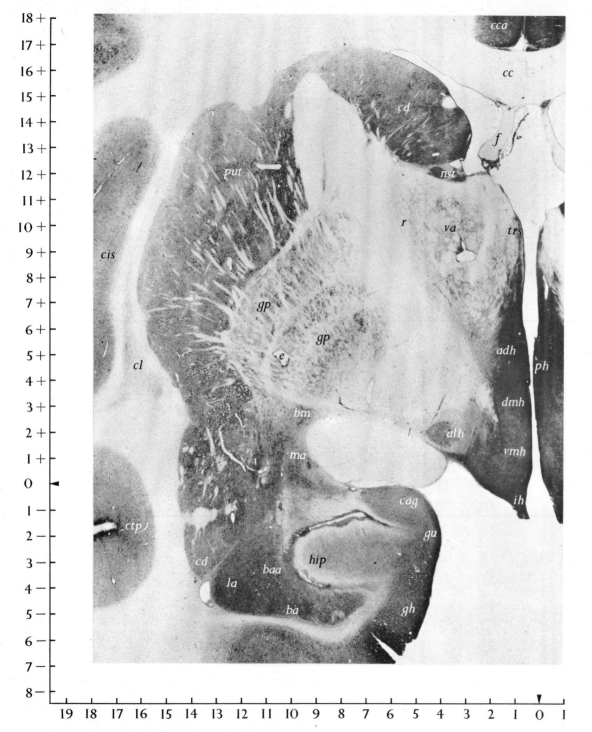

adh	Area dorsalis hypothalami
alh	Area lateralis hypothalami
ba	Nucleus basalis amygdalae
baa	Nucleus basalis accessorius amygdalae
bm	Nucleus basalis (Meynert)
cag	Nucleus corticalis amygdalae
cc	Corpus callosum
cca	Cortex cingularis anterior
cd	Nucleus caudatus
cis	Cortex insularis
cl	Claustrum
ctp	Cortex temporalis
dmh	Nucleus dorsalis medialis hypothalami
e	Electrode track
f	Fornix
gh	Gyrus hippocampi
gp	Globus pallidus
gu	Gyrus uncinatus
hip	Hippocampus
ih	Nucleus infundibularis hypothalami
la	Nucleus lateralis amygdalae
ma	Nucleus medialis amygdalae
nst	Nucleus striae terminalis
ph	Nucleus paraventricularis hypothalami
put	Putamen
r	Nucleus reticularis thalami
trs	Nucleus triangularis septi
va	Nucleus ventralis anterior thalami
vmh	Nucleus ventralis medialis hypothalami

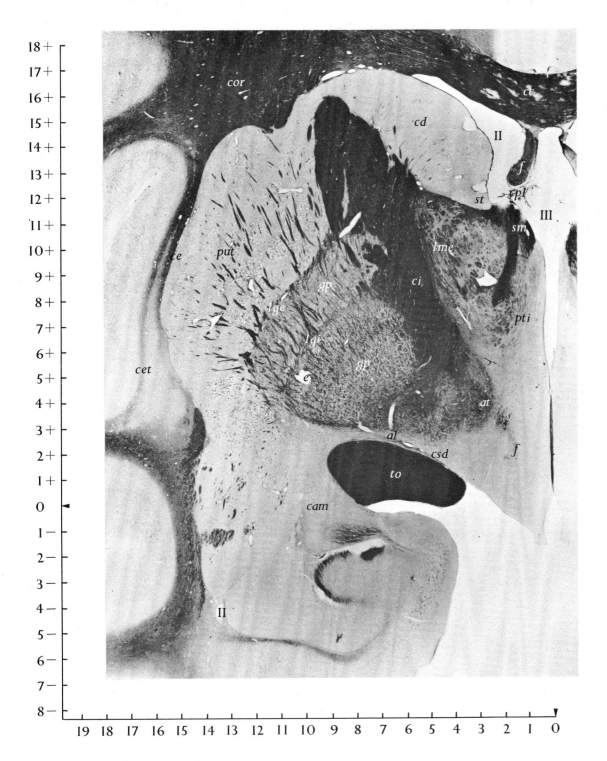

A 13·0 W

31

ad	Nucleus anterior dorsalis thalami
adh	Area dorsalis hypothalami
alh	Area lateralis hypothalami
av	Nucleus anterior ventralis thalami
ba	Nucleus basalis amygdalae
cc	Corpus callosum
cd	Nucleus caudatus
cis	Cortex insularis
cl	Claustrum
cpf	Cortex piriformis
cs	Nucleus centralis superior thalami
ctp	Cortex temporalis
dmh	Nucleus dorsalis medialis hypothalami
e	Electrode track
f	Fornix
gp	Globus pallidus
gph	Griseum periventriculare hypothalami
gu	Gyrus uncinatus
hip	Hippocampus
ih	Nucleus infundibularis hypothalami
la	Nucleus lateralis amygdalae
ma	Nucleus medialis amygdalae
md	Nucleus medialis dorsalis thalami
nst	Nucleus striae terminalis
pt	Nucleus parataenialis thalami
put	Putamen
r	Nucleus reticularis thalami
si	Substantia innominata
st	Stria terminalis
va	Nucleus ventralis anterior thalami
vmh	Nucleus ventralis medialis hypothalami
zi	Zona incerta

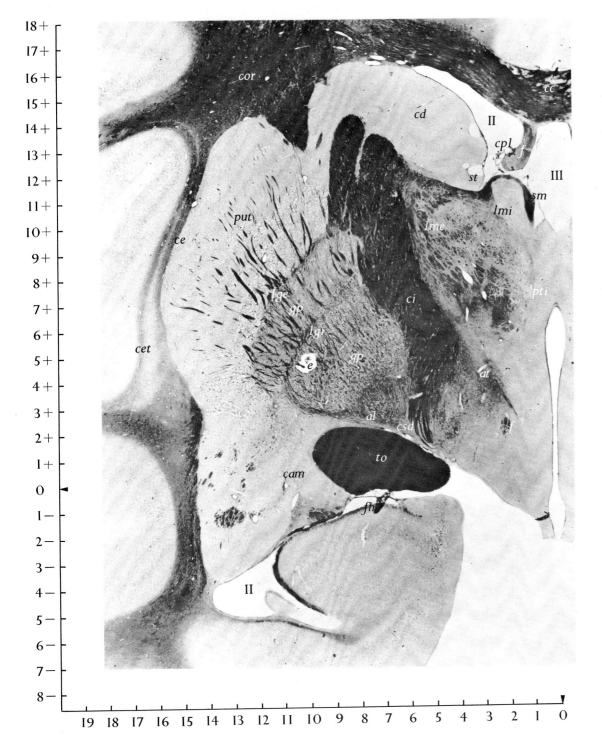

al	Ansa lenticularis
at	Area tegmentalis
cam	Corpus amygdalae
cc	Corpus callosum
cd	Nucleus caudatus
ce	Capsula externa
cet	Capsula extrema
ci	Capsula interna
cor	Corona radiata
cpl	Plexus choroidae ventriculi lateralis
csd	Commissura supraoptica dorsalis
e	Electrode track
f	Fornix
fh	Fimbria hippocampi
gp	Globus pallidus
lge	Globus pallidus, lamina medullaris externa
lgi	Globus pallidus, lamina medullaris interna
lme	Lamina medullaris externa thalami
lmi	Lamina medullaris interna thalami
pti	Pedunculus thalami inferior
put	Putamen
sm	Stria medullaris thalami
st	Stria terminalis
to	Tractus opticus
II	Ventriculus lateralis
III	Ventriculus tertius

33

ad   Nucleus anterior dorsalis thalami
adh   Area dorsalis hypothalami
alh   Area lateralis hypothalami
am   Nucleus anterior medialis thalami
av   Nucleus anterior ventralis thalami
cc   Corpus callosum
cd   Nucleus caudatus
cis   Cortex insularis
cl   Claustrum
cpf   Cortex piriformis
cs   Nucleus centralis superior thalami
ctp   Cortex temporalis
dmh   Nucleus dorsalis medialis hypothalami
e   Electrode track
em   Eminentia medialis
f   Fornix
gp   Globus pallidus
gph   Griseum periventriculare hypothalami
gu   Gyrus uncinatus
hip   Hippocampus
ma   Nucleus medialis amygdalae
md   Nucleus medialis dorsalis thalami
pt   Nucleus parataenialis thalami
put   Putamen
pv   Nucleus paraventricularis thalami
r   Nucleus reticularis thalami
ru   Nucleus reuniens thalami
si   Substantia innominata
st   Stria terminalis
va   Nucleus ventralis anterior thalami
vmh   Nucleus ventralis medialis hypothalami
zi   Zona incerta

34

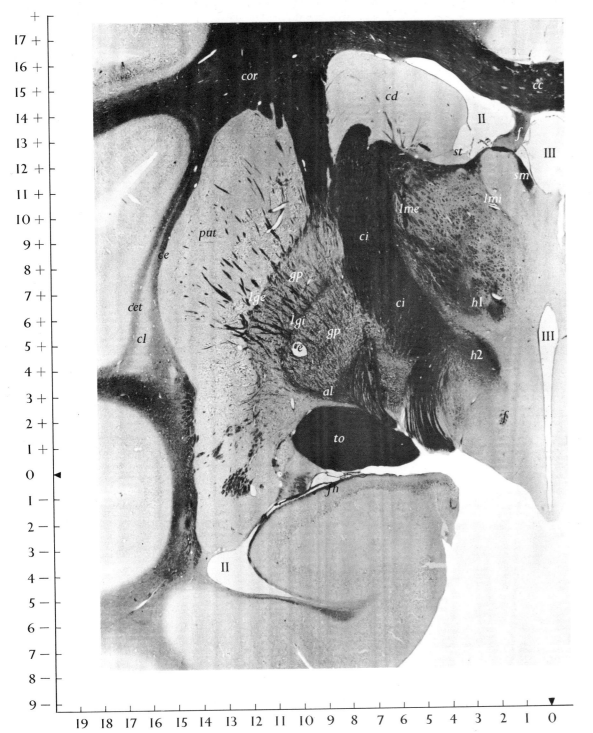

A 12·0 W

35

ad   Nucleus anterior dorsalis thalami
adh   Area dorsalis hypothalami
alh   Area lateralis hypothalami
am   Nucleus anterior medialis thalami
av   Nucleus anterior ventralis thalami
cc   Corpus callosum
cca   Cortex cingularis anterior
cd   Nucleus caudatus
cei   Nucleus centralis inferior thalami
cem   Nucleus centralis medialis thalami
cii   Nucleus centralis intermedius thalami
cis   Cortex insularis
cl   Claustrum
cpf   Cortex piriformis
cs   Nucleus centralis superior thalami
ctp   Cortex temporalis
e   Electrode track
f   Fornix
fd   Fascia dentata hippocampi
gp   Globus pallidus
gu   Gyrus uncinatus
hip   Hippocampus
md   Nucleus medialis dorsalis thalami
mi   Nucleus intermedius corpus mamillaris
ml   Nucleus lateralis corpus mamillaris
mm   Nucleus medialis corpus mamillaris
pt   Nucleus parataenialis thalami
put   Putamen
pv   Nucleus periventricularis thalami
r   Nucleus reticularis thalami
ru   Nucleus reuniens thalami
sbc   Subiculum
si   Substantia innominata
smt   Nucleus submedius thalami
st   Stria terminalis
va   Nucleus ventralis anterior thalami
vlo   Nucleus ventralis lateralis thalami, pars oralis
zi   Zona incerta

36

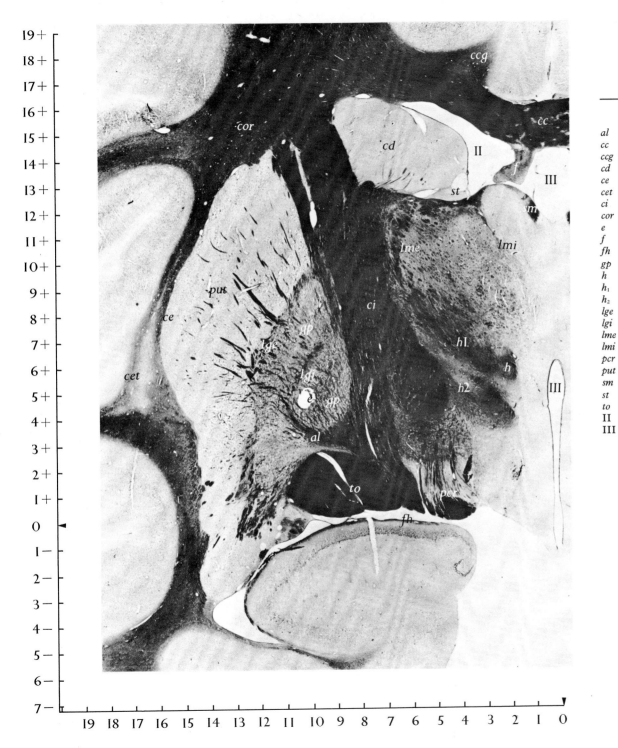

al	Ansa lenticularis
cc	Corpus callosum
ccg	Cingulum
cd	Nucleus caudatus
ce	Capsula externa
cet	Capsula extrema
ci	Capsula interna
cor	Corona radiata
e	Electrode track
f	Fornix
fh	Fimbria hippocampi
gp	Globus pallidus
h	Campus Foreli
h1	Campus Foreli, pars dorsalis
h2	Campus Foreli, pars ventralis
lge	Globus pallidus, lamina medullaris externa
lgi	Globus pallidus, lamina medullaris interna
lme	Lamina medullaris externa thalami
lmi	Lamina medullaris interna thalami
pcr	Pedunculus cerebri
put	Putamen
sm	Stria medullaris thalami
st	Stria terminalis
to	Tractus opticus
II	Ventriculus lateralis
III	Ventriculus tertius

37

A 11·0 C

ad Nucleus anterior dorsalis thalami
adh Area dorsalis hypothalami
alh Area lateralis hypothalami
am Nucleus anterior medialis thalami
av Nucleus anterior ventralis thalami
cc Corpus callosum
cca Cortex cingularis anterior
cd Nucleus caudatus
cei Nucleus centralis inferior thalami
cem Nucleus centralis medialis thalami
cii Nucleus centralis intermedius thalami
cis Cortex insularis
cl Claustrum
cpf Cortex piriformis
cs Nucleus centralis superior thalami
ctp Cortex temporalis
e Electrode track
f Fornix
fd Fascia dentata hippocampi
gp Globus pallidus
gu Gyrus uncinatus
hip Hippocampus
md Nucleus medialis dorsalis thalami
mi Nucleus intermedius corpus mamillaris
ml Nucleus lateralis corpus mamillaris
mm Nucleus medialis corpus mamillaris
pt Nucleus parataenialis thalami
put Putamen
pv Nucleus periventricularis thalami
r Nucleus reticularis thalami
ru Nucleus reuniens thalami
sbc Subiculum
si Substantia innominata
smt Nucleus submedius thalami
st Stria terminalis
va Nucleus ventralis anterior thalami
vlo Nucleus ventralis lateralis thalami, pars oralis
zi Zona incerta

38

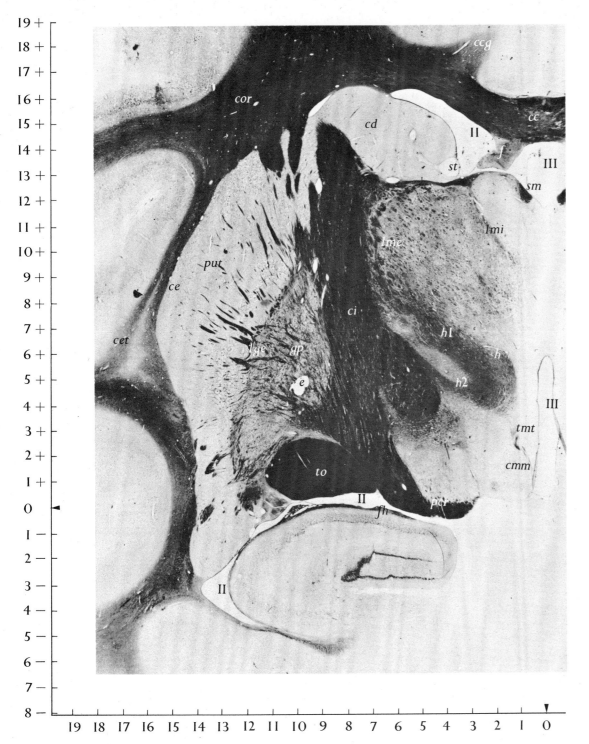

cc   Corpus callosum
ccg   Cingulum
cd   Nucleus caudatus
ce   Capsula externa
cet   Capsula extrema
ci   Capsula interna
cmm Corpus mamillare
cor   Corona radiata
e   Electrode track
f   Fornix
fh   Fimbria hippocampi
gp   Globus pallidus
h   Campus Foreli
h_1 Campus Foreli, pars dorsalis
h_2 Campus Foreli, pars ventralis
lge   Globus pallidus, lamina medullaris externa
lme   Lamina medullaris externa thalami
lmi   Lamina medullaris interna thalami
pcr   Pedunculus cerebri
put   Putamen
sm   Stria medullaris thalami
st   Stria terminalis
tmt   Tractus mamillothalamicus
to   Tractus opticus
II   Ventriculus lateralis
III   Ventriculus tertius

39

A 10·5 C

ad	Nucleus anterior dorsalis thalami
adh	Area dorsalis hypothalami
alh	Area lateralis hypothalami
am	Nucleus anterior medialis thalami
av	Nucleus anterior ventralis thalami
cc	Corpus callosum
cca	Cortex cingularis anterior
cd	Nucleus caudatus
cei	Nucleus centralis inferior thalami
cem	Nucleus centralis medialis thalami
cii	Nucleus centralis intermedius thalami
cis	Cortex insularis
cl	Claustrum
cpf	Cortex piriformis
cs	Nucleus centralis superior thalami
ctp	Cortex temporalis
e	Electrode track
f	Fornix
fd	Fascia dentata hippocampi
gp	Globus pallidus
gu	Gyrus uncinatus
hip	Hippocampus
md	Nucleus medialis dorsalis thalami
mi	Nucleus intermedius corpus mamillaris
ml	Nucleus lateralis corpus mamillaris
mm	Nucleus medialis corpus mamillaris
nsth	Nucleus subthalamicus
pt	Nucleus parataenialis thalami
put	Putamen
pv	Nucleus paraventricularis thalami
r	Nucleus reticularis thalami
ru	Nucleus reuniens thalami
sbc	Subiculum
smh	Nucleus supramamillaris hypothalami
smt	Nucleus submedius thalami
st	Stria terminalis
va	Nucleus ventralis anterior thalami
vlo	Nucleus ventralis lateralis thalami, pars oralis
zi	Zona incerta

40

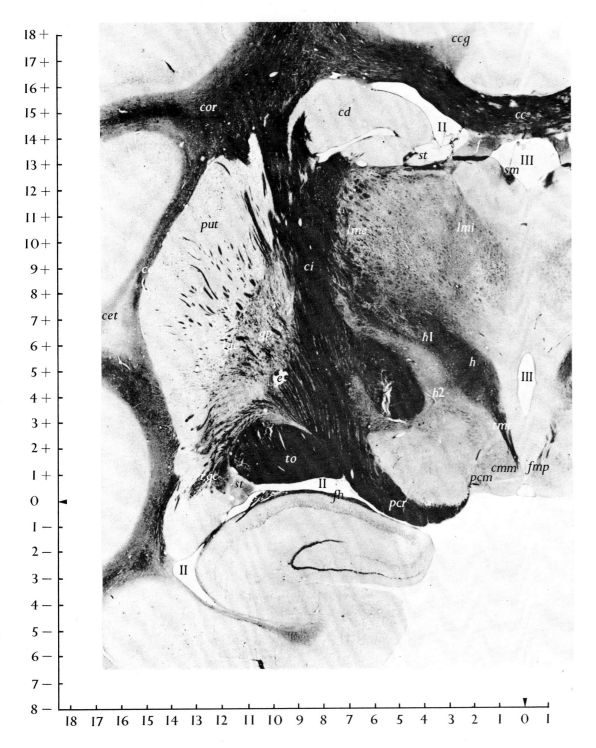

cc	Corpus callosum
ccg	Cingulum
cd	Nucleus caudatus
ce	Capsula externa
cet	Capsula extrema
ci	Capsula interna
cmm	Corpus mamillare
cor	Corona radiata
e	Electrode track
f	Fornix
fh	Fimbria hippocampi
fmp	Fasciculus mamillaris princeps
gp	Globus pallidus
h	Campus Foreli
h_1	Campus Foreli, pars dorsalis
h_2	Campus Foreli, pars ventralis
lge	Globus pallidus, lamina medullaris externa
lme	Lamina medullaris externa thalami
lmi	Lamina medullaris interna thalami
pcm	Pedunculus corporis mamillaris
pcr	Pedunculus cerebri
put	Putamen
rgc	Radiatio geniculo-calcarina
sm	Stria medullaris thalami
st	Stria terminalis
tmt	Tractus mamillothalamicus
to	Tractus opticus
II	Ventriculus lateralis
III	Ventriculus tertius

A 9·5 C

ad	Nucleus anterior dorsalis thalami
aph	Area posterior hypothalami
cc	Corpus callosum
cca	Cortex cingularis anterior
cd	Nucleus caudatus
cei	Nucleus centralis inferior thalami
cem	Nucleus centralis medialis thalami
cii	Nucleus centralis intermedius thalami
cpf	Cortex piriformis
cs	Nucleus centralis superior thalami
csl	Nucleus centralis superior lateralis thalami
e	Electrode track
f	Fornix
fd	Fascia dentata hippocampi
gh	Gyrus hippocampi
gl	Corpus geniculatum laterale
gp	Globus pallidus
gph	Griseum periventriculare hypothalami
gu	Gyrus uncinatus
hip	Hippocampus
ld	Nucleus lateralis dorsalis thalami
md	Nucleus medialis dorsalis thalami
nsth	Nucleus subthalamicus
pc	Nucleus paracentralis thalami
pt	Nucleus parataenialis thalami
put	Putamen
pv	Nucleus paraventricularis thalami
r	Nucleus reticularis thalami
sbc	Subiculum
smt	Nucleus submedius thalami
snc	Substantia nigra, pars compacta
snd	Substantia nigra, pars diffusa
st	Stria terminalis
vla	Nucleus ventralis lateralis thalami
vlm	Nucleus ventralis lateralis thalami, pars medialis
vlo	Nucleus ventralis lateralis thalami, pars oralis
zi	Zona incerta

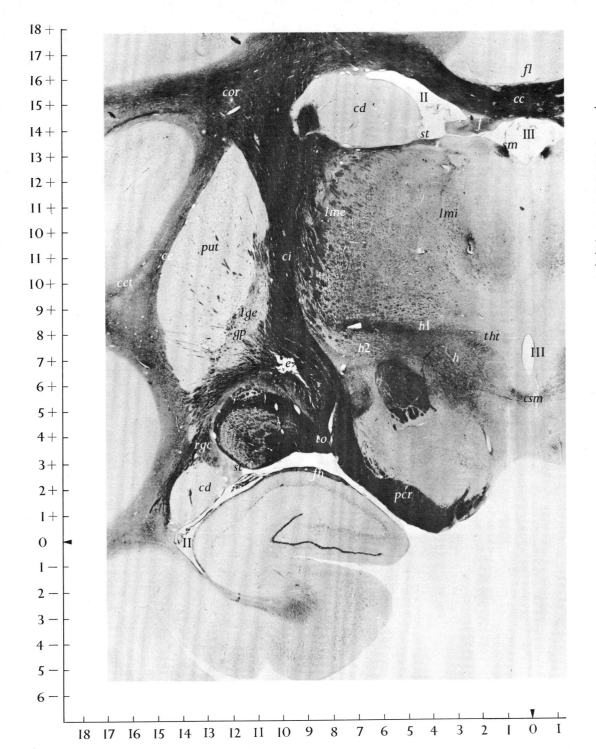

A 9·5 W

cc   Corpus callosum
cd   Nucleus caudatus
ce   Capsula externa
cet   Capsula extrema
ci   Capsula interna
cor   Corona radiata
csm   Commissura supramamillaris
e   Electrode track
f   Fornix
fh   Fimbria hippocampi
fl   Fissura longitudinalis cerebri
gp   Globus pallidus
h   Campus Foreli
h₁   Campus Foreli, pars dorsalis
h₂   Campus Foreli, pars ventralis
lge   Globus pallidus, lamina medullaris externa
lme   Lamina medullaris externa thalami
lmi   Lamina medullaris interna thalami
pcr   Pedunculus cerebri
put   Putamen
rgc   Radiatio geniculo-calcarina
sm   Stria medullaris thalami
st   Stria terminalis
tht   Tractus hypothalamicotegmentalis
to   Tractus opticus
II   Ventriculus lateralis
III   Ventriculus tertius

43

ad	Nucleus anterior dorsalis thalami
cc	Corpus callosum
cca	Cortex cingularis
cd	Nucleus caudatus
cei	Nucleus centralis inferior thalami
cem	Nucleus centralis medialis thalami
cm	Centrum medianum thalami
cpf	Cortex piriformis
cs	Nucleus centralis superior thalami
csl	Nucleus centralis superior lateralis thalami
e	Electrode track
f	Fornix
fd	Fascia dentata hippocampi
fh	Fimbria hippocampi
gh	Gyrus hippocampi
gl	Corpus geniculatum laterale
gpm	Griseum periventriculare mesencephali
gu	Gyrus uncinatus
hip	Hippocampus
ip	Nucleus interpeduncularis
ld	Nucleus lateralis dorsalis thalami
md	Nucleus medialis dorsalis thalami
nr	Nucleus ruber
nsth	Nucleus subthalamicus
pc	Nucleus paracentralis thalami
put	Putamen
pv	Nucleus paraventricularis thalami
r	Nucleus reticularis thalami
sbc	Subiculum
smt	Nucleus submedius thalami
snc	Substantia nigra, pars compacta
snd	Substantia nigra, pars diffusa
st	Stria terminalis
vla	Nucleus ventralis lateralis thalami
vlo	Nucleus ventralis lateralis thalami, pars oralis
vpi	Nucleus ventralis posterior inferior thalami
vpl	Nucleus ventralis posterior lateralis thalami
vpm	Nucleus ventralis posterior medialis thalami
zi	Zona incerta

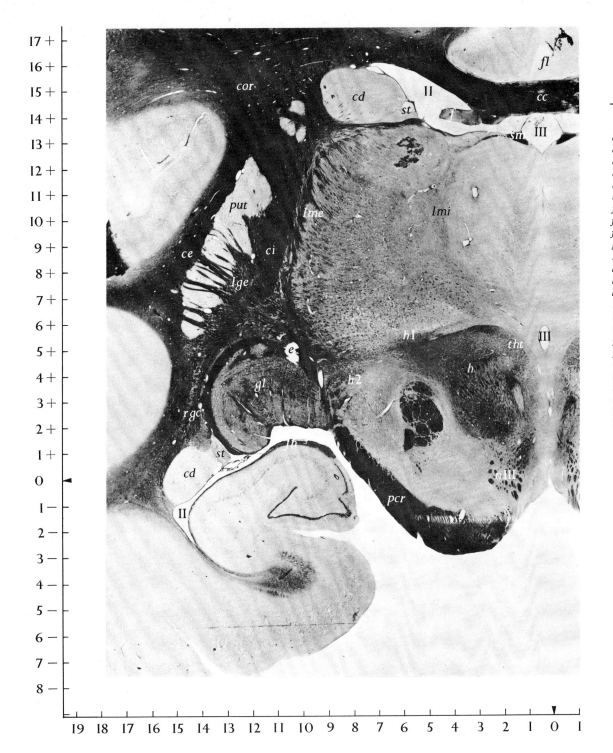

cc	Corpus callosum
cd	Nucleus caudatus
ce	Capsula externa
ci	Capsula interna
cor	Corona radiata
e	Electrode track
f	Fornix
fh	Fimbria hippocampi
fl	Fissura longitudinalis cerebri
gl	Corpus geniculatum laterale
h	Campus Foreli
h_1	Campus Foreli, pars dorsalis
h_2	Campus Foreli, pars ventralis
lge	Globus pallidus, lamina medullaris externa
lme	Lamina medullaris externa thalami
lmi	Lamina medullaris interna thalami
nIII	Nervus oculomotorius
pcr	Pedunculus cerebri
put	Putamen
rgc	Radiatio geniculo-calcarina
sm	Stria medullaris thalami
st	Stria terminalis
tht	Tractus hypothalamicotegmentalis
II	Ventriculus lateralis
III	Ventriculus tertius

A 8·0 C

ad	Nucleus anterior dorsalis thalami
cc	Corpus callosum
cca	Cortex cingularis
cd	Nucleus caudatus
cei	Nucleus centralis inferior thalami
cel	Nucleus centralis lateralis thalami
cm	Centrum medianum thalami
cpf	Cortex piriformis
cs	Nucleus centralis superior thalami
csl	Nucleus centralis superior lateralis thalami
e	Electrode track
f	Fornix
fd	Fascia dentata hippocampi
frtm	Formatio reticularis tegmenti mesencephali
gh	Gyrus hippocampi
gl	Corpus geniculatum laterale
gpm	Griseum periventriculare mesencephali
hip	Hippocampus
ip	Nucleus interpeduncularis
ld	Nucleus lateralis dorsalis thalami
lp	Nucleus lateralis posterior thalami
md	Nucleus medialis dorsalis thalami
ndk	Nucleus Darkschewitsch
now	Nucleus rostralis n. oculomotorii (Westphal–Edinger)
nr	Nucleus ruber
nsth	Nucleus subthalamicus
pf	Nucleus parafascicularis thalami
put	Putamen
pv	Nucleus paraventricularis thalami
r	Nucleus reticularis thalami
smt	Nucleus submedius thalami
sn	Substantia nigra
st	Stria terminalis
vla	Nucleus ventralis lateralis thalami
vpi	Nucleus ventralis posterior inferior thalami
vpl	Nucleus ventralis posterior lateralis thalami
vpm	Nucleus ventralis posterior medialis thalami
zi	Zona incerta

46

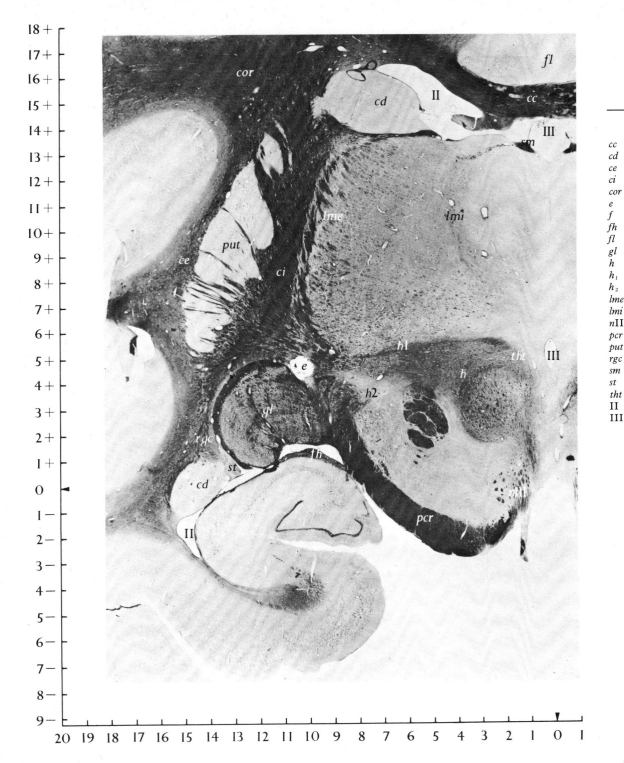

A 8·0 W

cc	Corpus callosum
cd	Nucleus caudatus
ce	Capsula externa
ci	Capsula interna
cor	Corona radiata
e	Electrode track
f	Fornix
fh	Fimbria hippocampi
fl	Fissura longitudinalis cerebri
gl	Corpus geniculatum laterale
h	Campus Foreli
h_1	Campus Foreli, pars dorsalis
h_2	Campus Foreli, pars ventralis
lme	Lamina medullaris externa thalami
lmi	Lamina medullaris interna thalami
nIII	Nervus oculomotorius
pcr	Pedunculus cerebri
put	Putamen
rgc	Radiatio geniculo-calcarina
sm	Stria medullaris thalami
st	Stria terminalis
tht	Tractus hypothalamicotegmentalis
II	Ventriculus lateralis
III	Ventriculus tertius

47

ad	Nucleus anterior dorsalis thalami
cc	Corpus callosum
cca	Cortex cingularis
cd	Nucleus caudatus
cei	Nucleus centralis inferior thalami
cel	Nucleus centralis lateralis thalami
cm	Centrum medianum thalami
cpf	Cortex piriformis
cs	Nucleus centralis superior thalami
csl	Nucleus centralis superior lateralis thalami
e	Electrode track
f	Fornix
fd	Fascia dentata hippocampi
frtm	Formatio reticularis tegmenti mesencephali
fs	Fissura lateralis cerebri (Sylvii)
gh	Gyrus hippocampi
gl	Corpus geniculatum laterale
glo	Corpus geniculatum laterale, pars oralis
gm	Corpus geniculatum mediale
gpm	Griseum periventriculare mesencephali
hip	Hippocampus
ip	Nucleus interpeduncularis
is	Nucleus interstitialis (Cajal)
ld	Nucleus lateralis dorsalis thalami
lp	Nucleus lateralis posterior thalami
md	Nucleus medialis dorsalis thalami
noc	Nucleus centralis n. oculomotorii
nod	Nucleus n. oculomotorii, pars dorsalis
nov	Nucleus n. oculomotorii, pars ventralis
nr	Nucleus ruber
pd	Nucleus peripeduncularis thalami
pf	Nucleus parafascicularis thalami
put	Putamen
pv	Nucleus paraventricularis thalami
r	Nucleus reticularis thalami
sn	Substantia nigra
st	Stria terminalis
vpi	Nucleus ventralis posterior inferior thalami
vpl	Nucleus ventralis posterior lateralis thalami
vpm	Nucleus ventralis posterior medialis thalami

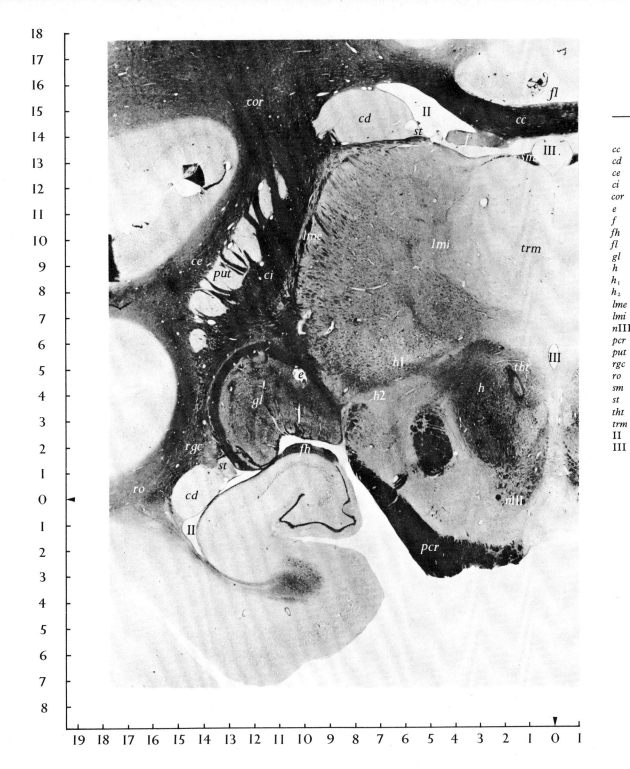

cc	Corpus callosum
cd	Nucleus caudatus
ce	Capsula externa
ci	Capsula interna
cor	Corona radiata
e	Electrode track
f	Fornix
fh	Fimbria hippocampi
fl	Fissura longitudinalis cerebri
gl	Corpus geniculatum laterale
h	Campus Foreli
h₁	Campus Foreli, pars dorsalis
h₂	Campus Foreli, pars ventralis
lme	Lamina medullaris externa thalami
lmi	Lamina medullaris interna thalami
nIII	Nervus oculomotorius
pcr	Pedunculus cerebri
put	Putamen
rgc	Radiatio geniculo-calcarina
ro	Radiatio optica
sm	Stria medullaris thalami
st	Stria terminalis
tht	Tractus hypothalamicotegmentalis
trm	Tractus retroflexus (Meynert)
II	Ventriculus lateralis
III	Ventriculus tertius

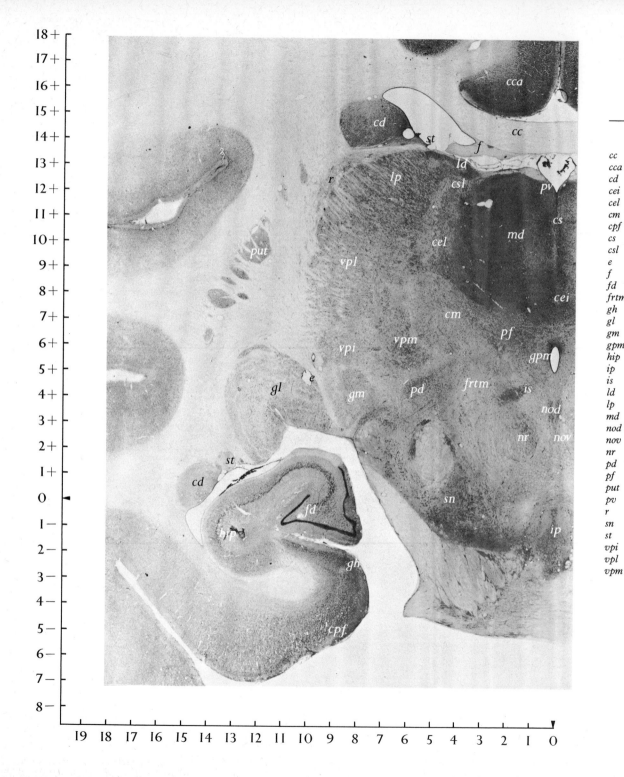

A 7·0 C

cc	Corpus callosum
cca	Cortex cingularis
cd	Nucleus caudatus
cei	Nucleus centralis inferior thalami
cel	Nucleus centralis lateralis thalami
cm	Centrum medianum thalami
cpf	Cortex piriformis
cs	Nucleus centralis superior thalami
csl	Nucleus centralis superior lateralis thalami
e	Electrode track
f	Fornix
fd	Fascia dentata hippocampi
frtm	Formatio reticularis tegmenti mesencephali
gh	Gyrus hippocampi
gl	Corpus geniculatum laterale
gm	Corpus geniculatum mediale
gpm	Griseum periventriculare mesencephali
hip	Hippocampus
ip	Nucleus interpeduncularis
is	Nucleus interstitialis (Cajal)
ld	Nucleus lateralis dorsalis thalami
lp	Nucleus lateralis posterior thalami
md	Nucleus medialis dorsalis thalami
nod	Nucleus n. oculomotorii, pars dorsalis
nov	Nucleus n. oculomotorii, pars ventralis
nr	Nucleus ruber
pd	Nucleus peripeduncularis thalami
pf	Nucleus parafascicularis thalami
put	Putamen
pv	Nucleus paraventricularis thalami
r	Nucleus reticularis thalami
sn	Substantia nigra
st	Stria terminalis
vpi	Nucleus ventralis posterior inferior thalami
vpl	Nucleus ventralis posterior lateralis thalami
vpm	Nucleus ventralis posterior medialis thalami

50

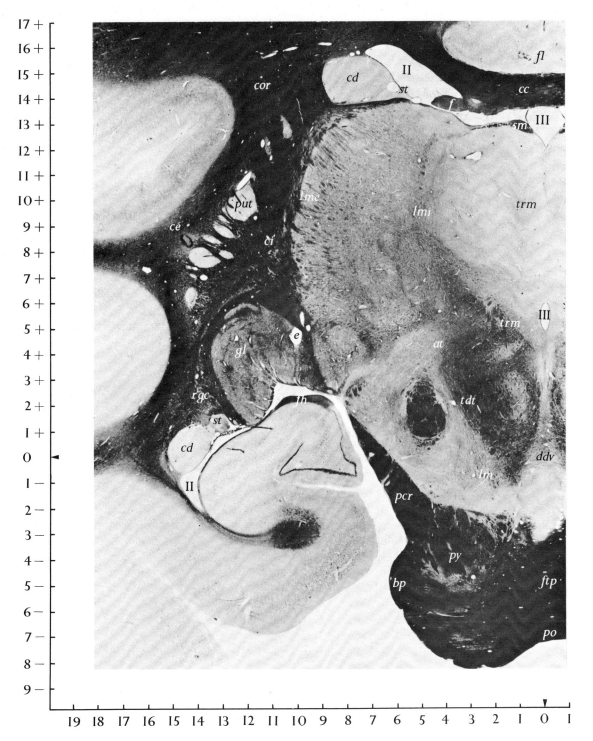

at	Area tegmentalis
bp	Brachium pontis
cc	Corpus callosum
cd	Nucleus caudatus
ce	Capsula externa
ci	Capsula interna
cor	Corona radiata
ddv	Decussatio ventralis tegmenti
e	Electrode track
f	Fornix
fh	Fimbria hippocampi
fl	Fissura longitudinalis cerebri
ftp	Fibrae pontis transversae
gl	Corpus geniculatum laterale
lm	Lemniscus medialis
lme	Lamina medullaris externa thalami
lmi	Lamina medullaris interna thalami
pcr	Pedunculus cerebri
po	Pons
put	Putamen
py	Tractus pyramidalis
rgc	Radiatio geniculo-calcarina
sm	Stria medullaris thalami
st	Stria terminalis
tdt	Tractus dentatothalamicus
trm	Tractus retroflexus (Meynert)
II	Ventriculus lateralis
III	Ventriculus tertius

51

an	Nucleus annularis
cc	Corpus callosum
cca	Cortex cingularis
cd	Nucleus caudatus
cei	Nucleus centralis inferior thalami
cel	Nucleus centralis lateralis thalami
cm	Centrum medianum thalami
cpf	Cortex piriformis
cs	Nucleus centralis superior thalami
csl	Nucleus centralis superior lateralis thalami
e	Electrode track
f	Fornix
fd	Fascia dentata hippocampi
frtm	Formatio reticularis tegmenti mesencephali
gl	Corpus geniculatum laterale
gm	Corpus geniculatum mediale
gpm	Griseum periventriculare mesencephali
gpo	Griseum pontis
hip	Hippocampus
ip	Nucleus interpeduncularis
ld	Nucleus lateralis dorsalis thalami
lp	Nucleus lateralis posterior thalami
md	Nucleus medialis dorsalis thalami
noc	Nucleus centralis n. oculomotorii
nod	Nucleus n. oculomotorii, pars dorsalis
nov	Nucleus n. oculomotorii, pars ventralis
nr	Nucleus ruber
pd	Nucleus peripeduncularis thalami
pf	Nucleus parafascicularis thalami
put	Putamen
pv	Nucleus paraventricularis thalami
pvo	Nucleus pulvinaris oralis thalami
r	Nucleus reticularis thalami
rtp	Nucleus reticularis tegmenti pontis
sn	Substantia nigra
st	Stria terminalis
vpi	Nucleus ventralis posterior inferior thalami
vpl	Nucleus ventralis posterior lateralis thalami
vpm	Nucleus ventralis posterior medialis thalami

52

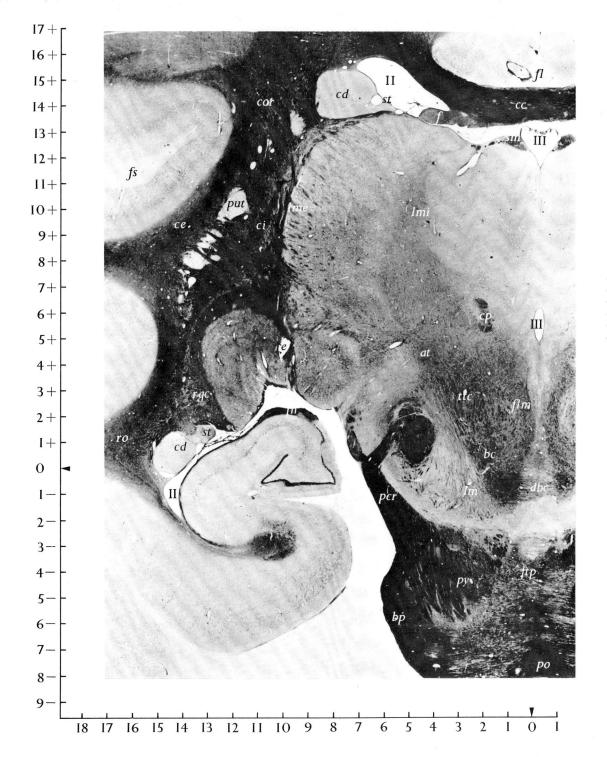

A 6·5 W

A 6·0 C

an	Nucleus annularis
cc	Corpus callosum
cca	Cortex cingularis
cd	Nucleus caudatus
cei	Nucleus centralis inferior thalami
cel	Nucleus centralis lateralis thalami
cm	Centrum medianum thalami
cs	Nucleus centralis superior thalami
csl	Nucleus centralis superior lateralis thalami
e	Electrode track
f	Fornix
fd	Fascia dentata hippocampi
fh	Fimbria hippocampi
frtm	Formatio reticularis tegmenti mesencephali
gh	Gyrus hippocampi
gl	Corpus geniculatum laterale
gm	Corpus geniculatum mediale
gpm	Griseum periventriculare mesencephali
gpo	Griseum pontis
hip	Hippocampus
ip	Nucleus interpeduncularis
ld	Nucleus lateralis dorsalis thalami
lp	Nucleus lateralis posterior thalami
md	Nucleus medialis dorsalis thalami
noc	Nucleus centralis n. oculomotorii
nod	Nucleus n. oculomotorii, pars dorsalis
nov	Nucleus n. oculomotorii, pars ventralis
nr	Nucleus ruber
pf	Nucleus parafascicularis thalami
put	Putamen
pv	Nucleus paraventricularis thalami
pvo	Nucleus pulvinaris oralis thalami
r	Nucleus reticularis thalami
rtp	Nucleus reticularis tegmenti pontis
sn	Substantia nigra
st	Stria terminalis
vpl	Nucleus ventralis posterior lateralis thalami
vpm	Nucleus ventralis posterior medialis thalami

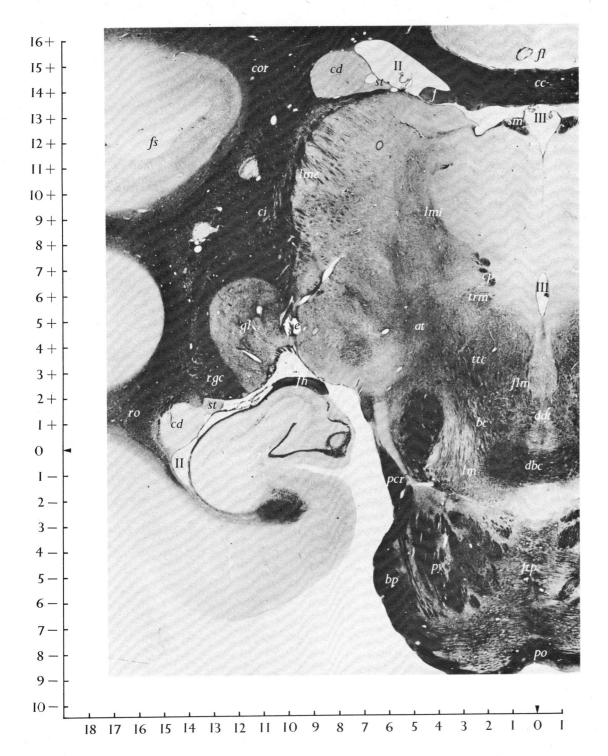

at	Area tegmentalis
bc	Brachium conjunctivum
bp	Brachium pontis
cc	Corpus callosum
cd	Nucleus caudatus
ci	Capsula interna
cor	Corona radiata
cp	Commissura posterior
dbc	Decussatio brachii conjunctivi
ddt	Decussatio dorsalis tegmenti
e	Electrode track
f	Fornix
fh	Fimbria hippocampi
fl	Fissura longitudinalis cerebri
flm	Fasciculus longitudinalis medialis
fs	Fissura lateralis cerebri (Sylvii)
ftp	Fibrae pontis transversae
gl	Corpus geniculatum laterale
lm	Lemniscus medialis
lme	Lamina medullaris externa thalami
lmi	Lamina medullaris interna thalami
pcr	Pedunculus cerebri
po	Pons
py	Tractus pyramidalis
rgc	Radiatio geniculo-calcarina
ro	Radiatio optica
sm	Stria medullaris thalami
st	Stria terminalis
trm	Tractus retroflexus (Meynert)
ttc	Tractus tegmentalis centralis
II	Ventriculus lateralis
III	Ventriculus tertius

55

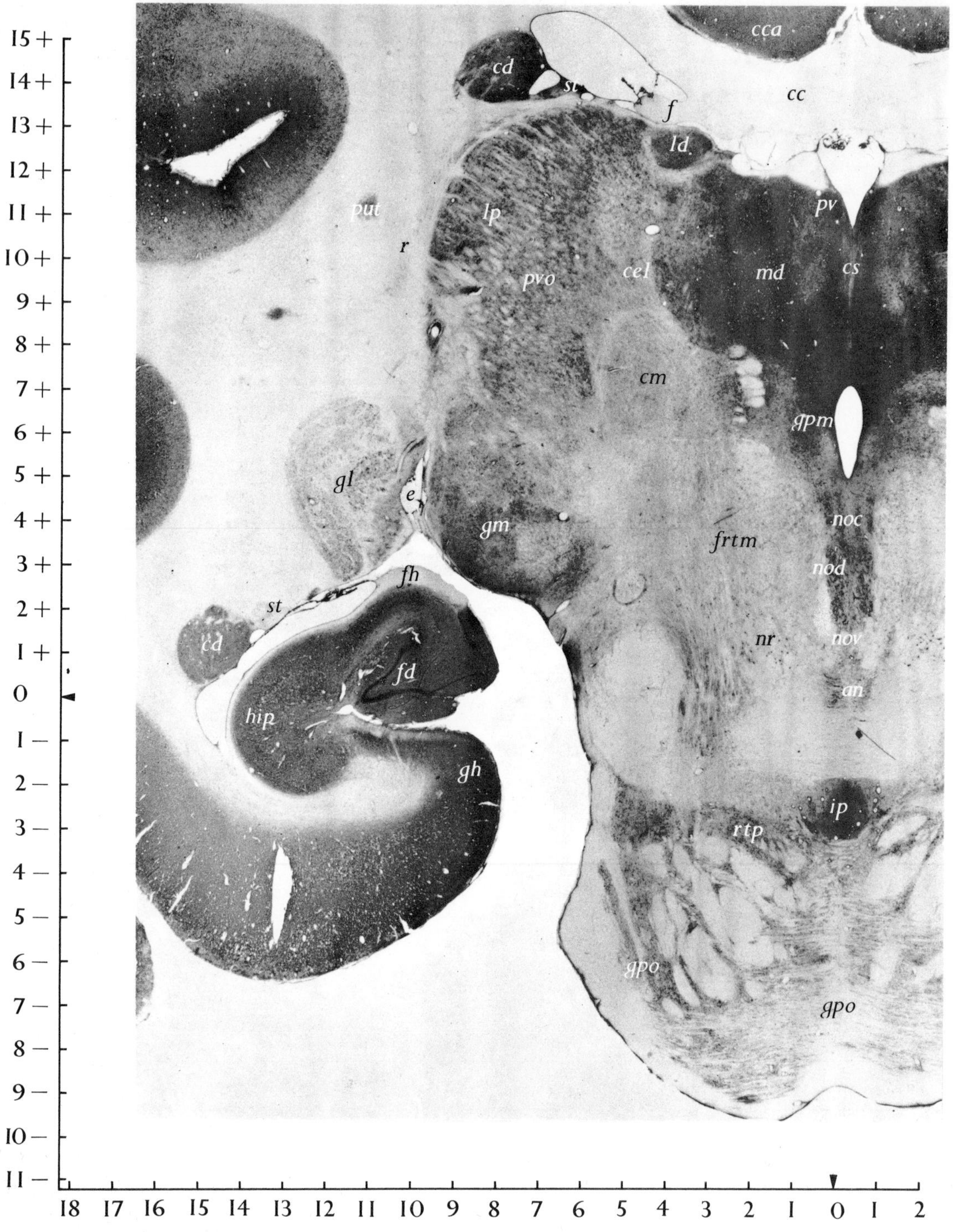

15+
14+
13+
12+
11+
10+
9+
8+
7+
6+
5+
4+
3+
2+
1+
0
1−
2−
3−
4−
5−
6−
7−
8−
9−
10−
11−

18 17 16 15 14 13 12 11 10 9 8 7 6 5 4 3 2 1 0 1 2

Labels on section: cca, cd, st, cc, f, ld, pv, put, lp, r, pvo, cel, md, cs, cm, gpm, gl, e, gm, frtm, noc, nod, nov, an, fh, st, cd, fd, hip, gh, nr, ip, rtp, gpo, gpo

an	Nucleus annularis
cc	Corpus callosum
cca	Cortex cingularis
cd	Nucleus caudatus
cel	Nucleus centralis lateralis thalami
cm	Centrum medianum thalami
cs	Nucleus centralis superior thalami
e	Electrode track
f	Fornix
fd	Fascia dentata hippocampi
fh	Fimbria hippocampi
frtm	Formatio reticularis tegmenti mesencephali
gh	Gyrus hippocampi
gl	Corpus geniculatum laterale
gm	Corpus geniculatum mediale
gpm	Griseum periventriculare mesencephali
gpo	Griseum pontis
hip	Hippocampus
ip	Nucleus interpeduncularis
ld	Nucleus lateralis dorsalis thalami
lp	Nucleus lateralis posterior thalami
md	Nucleus medialis dorsalis thalami
noc	Nucleus centralis n. oculomotorii
nod	Nucleus n. oculomotorii, pars dorsalis
nov	Nucleus n. oculomotorii, pars ventralis
nr	Nucleus ruber
put	Putamen
pv	Nucleus paraventricularis thalami
pvo	Nucleus pulvinaris oralis thalami
r	Nucleus reticularis thalami
rtp	Nucleus reticularis tegmenti pontis
st	Stria terminalis

56

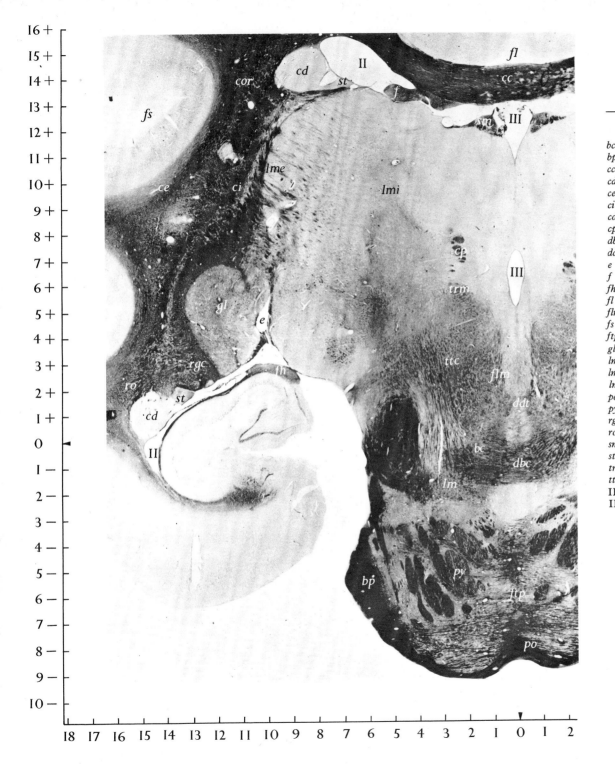

bc   Brachium conjunctivum
bp   Brachium pontis
cc   Corpus callosum
cd   Nucleus caudatus
ce   Capsula externa
ci   Capsula interna
cor Corona radiata
cp   Commissura posterior
dbc Decussatio brachii conjunctivi
ddt Decussatio dorsalis tegmenti
e   Electrode track
f   Fornix
fh   Fimbria hippocampi
fl   Fasciculus longitudinalis cerebri
flm Fasciculus longitudinalis medialis
fs   Fissura lateralis cerebri (Sylvii)
ftp Fibrae pontis transversae
gl   Corpus geniculatum laterale
lm   Lemniscus medialis
lme Lamina medullaris externa thalami
lmi Lamina medullaris interna thalami
po   Pons
py   Tractus pyramidalis
rgc Radiatio geniculo-calcarina
ro   Radiatio optica
sm   Stria medullaris thalami
st   Stria terminalis
trm Tractus retroflexus (Meynert)
ttc Tractus tegmentalis centralis
II   Ventriculus lateralis
III Ventriculus tertius

A 4·5 C

an   Nucleus annularis
apt   Area praetectalis
cc   Corpus callosum
cd   Nucleus caudatus
e   Electrode track
f   Fornix
fd   Fascia dentata hippocampi
fh   Fimbria hippocampi
fl   Fissura longitudinalis cerebri
frtm   Formatio reticularis tegmenti mesencephali
gc   Substantia grisea centralis
gh   Gyrus hippocampi
gm   Corpus geniculatum mediale
gmm   Corpus geniculatum mediale, pars magnocellularis
gpo   Griseum pontis
hip   Hippocampus
hl   Nucleus habenularis lateralis epithalami
hm   Nucleus habenularis medialis epithalami
ip   Nucleus interpeduncularis
lmt   Nucleus limitans thalami
md   Nucleus medialis dorsalis thalami
noc   Nucleus centralis n. oculomotorii
nod   Nucleus n. oculomotorii, pars dorsalis
nov   Nucleus n. oculomotorii, pars ventralis
put   Putamen
pvi   Nucleus pulvinaris inferior thalami
pvl   Nucleus pulvinaris lateralis thalami
pvm   Nucleus pulvinaris medialis thalami
r   Nucleus reticularis thalami
rtp   Nucleus reticularis tegmenti pontis
st   Stria terminalis

58

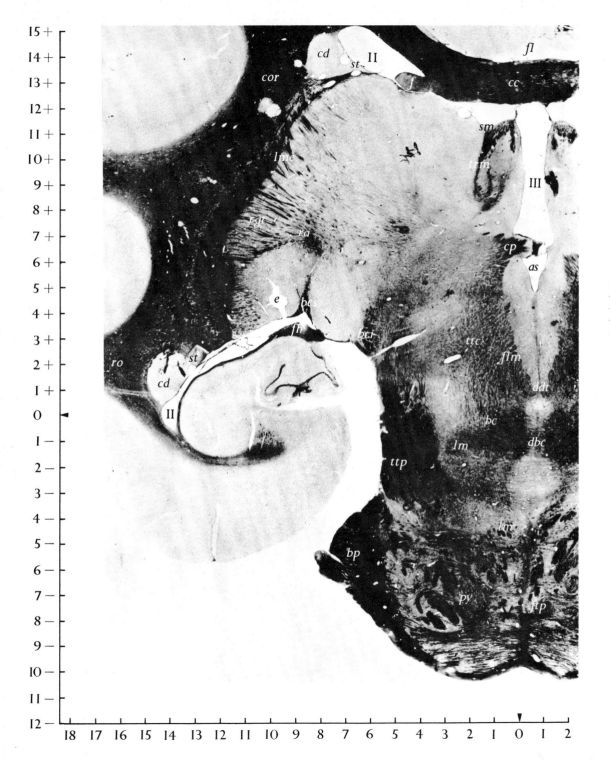

A 4·5 W

as	Aquaeductus Sylvii
bc	Brachium conjunctivum
bci	Brachium colliculi inferioris
bcs	Brachium colliculi superioris
bp	Brachium pontis
cc	Corpus callosum
cd	Nucleus caudatus
cor	Corona radiata
cp	Commissura posterior
dbc	Decussatio brachii conjunctivi
ddt	Decussatio dorsalis tegmenti
e	Electrode track
f	Fornix
fh	Fimbria hippocampi
fl	Fissura longitudinalis cerebri
flm	Fasciculus longitudinalis medialis
ftp	Fibrae pontis transversae
lm	Lemniscus medialis
lme	Lamina medullaris externa thalami
py	Tractus pyramidalis
ra	Radiatio acustica
rgt	Radiatio geniculo-temporalis
ro	Radiatio optica
sm	Stria medullaris thalami
st	Stria terminalis
trm	Tractus retroflexus (Meynert)
ttc	Tractus tegmentalis centralis
ttp	Tractus tectopontinus
II	Ventriculus lateralis
III	Ventriculus tertius

59

A 3·5 C

an   Nucleus annularis
apt   Area praetectalis
cc   Corpus callosum
cca   Cortex cingularis
cd   Nucleus caudatus
e   Electrode track
f   Fornix
fd   Fascia dentata hippocampi
fh   Fimbria hippocampi
fl   Fissura longitudinalis cerebri
frp   Formatio reticularis pontis
frtm Formatio reticularis tegmenti mesencephali
gc   Substantia grisea centralis
gh   Gyrus hippocampi
gm   Corpus geniculatum mediale
gpo   Griseum pontis
hip   Hippocampus
hl   Nucleus habenularis lateralis epithalami
hm   Nucleus habenularis medialis epithalami
ip   Nucleus interpeduncularis
lmt   Nucleus limitans thalami
md   Nucleus medialis dorsalis thalami
noc   Nucleus centralis n. oculomotorii
nod   Nucleus n. oculomotorii, pars dorsalis
nov   Nucleus n. oculomotorii, pars ventralis
pvi   Nucleus pulvinaris inferior thalami
pvl   Nucleus pulvinaris lateralis thalami
pvm   Nucleus pulvinaris medialis thalami
r   Nucleus reticularis thalami
rtp   Nucleus reticularis tegmenti pontis
st   Stria terminalis

60

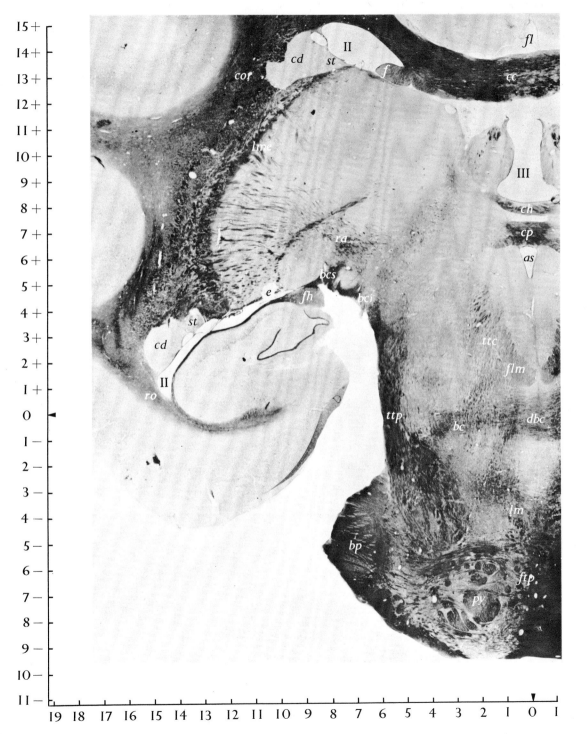

A 3·5 W

as	Aquaeductus Sylvii
bc	Brachium conjunctivum
bci	Brachium colliculi inferioris
bcs	Brachium colliculi superioris
bp	Brachium pontis
cc	Corpus callosum
cd	Nucleus caudatus
ch	Commissura habenulae
cor	Corona radiata
cp	Commissura posterior
dbc	Decussatio brachii conjunctivi
e	Electrode track
f	Fornix
fh	Fimbria hippocampi
fl	Fissura longitudinalis cerebri
flm	Fasciculus longitudinalis medialis
ftp	Fibrae pontis transversae
lm	Lemniscus medialis
lme	Lamina medullaris externa thalami
py	Tractus pyramidalis
ra	Radiatio acustica
ro	Radiatio optica
st	Stria terminalis
ttc	Tractus tegmentalis centralis
ttp	Tractus tectopontinus
II	Ventriculus lateralis
III	Ventriculus tertius

61

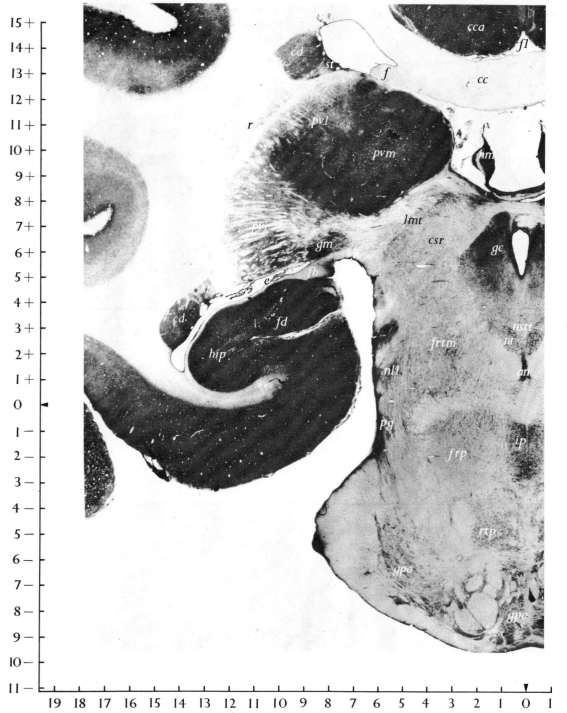

an	Nucleus annularis
cc	Corpus callosum
cca	Cortex cingularis
cd	Nucleus caudatus
csr	Colliculus superior
e	Electrode track
f	Fornix
fd	Fascia dentata hippocampi
fh	Fimbria hippocampi
fl	Fissura longitudinalis cerebri
frp	Formatio reticularis pontis
frtm	Formatio reticularis tegmenti mesencephali
gc	Substantia grisea centralis
gm	Corpus geniculatum mediale
gpo	Griseum pontis
hip	Hippocampus
hm	Nucleus habenularis medialis epithalami
ip	Nucleus interpeduncularis
lmt	Nucleus limitans thalami
nll	Nucleus lemnisci lateralis
nstt	Nucleus supratrochlearis
nt	Nucleus n. trochlearis
pg	Nucleus parabigeminalis
pvi	Nucleus pulvinaris inferior thalami
pvl	Nucleus pulvinaris lateralis thalami
pvm	Nucleus pulvinaris medialis thalami
r	Nucleus reticularis thalami
rtp	Nucleus reticularis tegmenti pontis
st	Stria terminalis

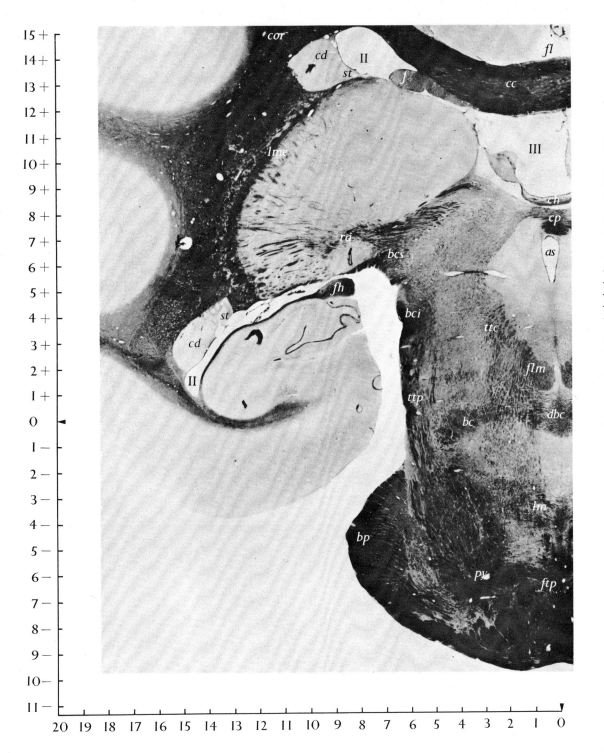

A 3·0 W

as	Aquaeductus Sylvii
bc	Brachium conjunctivum
bci	Brachium colliculi inferioris
bcs	Brachium colliculi superioris
bp	Brachium pontis
cc	Corpus callosum
cd	Nucleus caudatus
ch	Commissura habenulae
cor	Corona radiata
cp	Commissura posterior
dbc	Decussatio brachii conjunctivi
f	Fornix
fh	Fimbria hippocampi
fl	Fissura longitudinalis cerebri
flm	Fasciculus longitudinalis medialis
ftp	Fibrae pontis transversae
lm	Lemniscus medialis
lme	Lamina medullaris externa thalami
py	Tractus pyramidalis
ra	Radiatio acustica
st	Stria terminalis
ttc	Tractus tegmentalis centralis
ttp	Tractus tectopontinus
II	Ventriculus lateralis
III	Ventriculus tertius

63

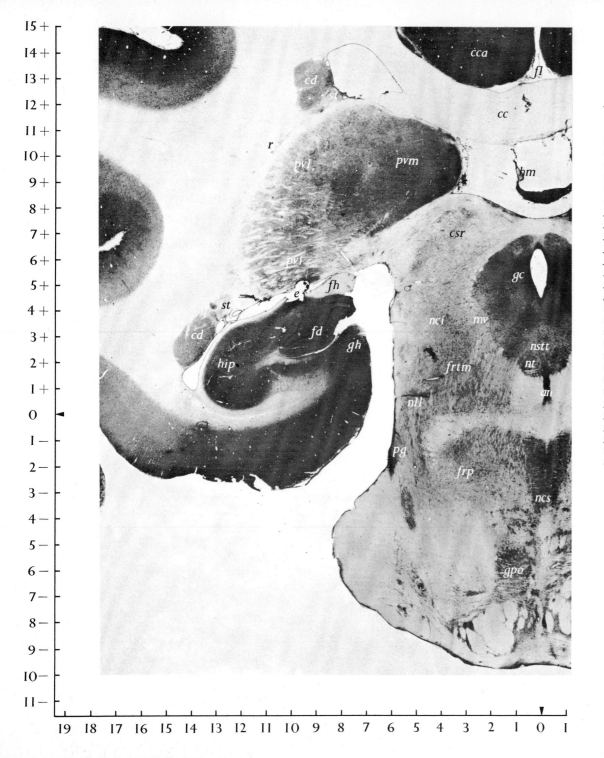

A 2·5 C

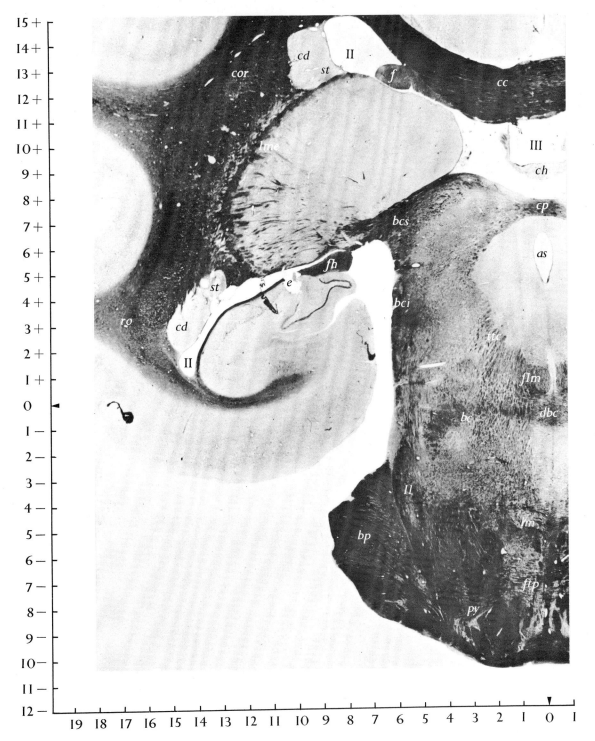

A 2·5 W

as   Aquaeductus Sylvii
bc   Brachium conjunctivum
bci   Brachium colliculi inferioris
bcs   Brachium colliculi superioris
bp   Brachium pontis
cc   Corpus callosum
cd   Nucleus caudatus
ch   Commissura habenulae
cor   Corona radiata
cp   Commissura posterior
dbc   Decussatio brachii conjunctivi
e   Electrode track
f   Fornix
fh   Fimbria hippocampi
flm   Fasciculus longitudinalis medialis
ftp   Fibrae pontis transversae
ll   Lemniscus lateralis
lm   Lemniscus medialis
lme   Lamina medullaris externa thalami
py   Tractus pyramidalis
ro   Radiatio optica
st   Stria terminalis
ttc   Tractus tegmentalis centralis
II   Ventriculus lateralis
III   Ventriculus tertius

65

A 2·0 C

an   Nucleus annularis
cc   Corpus callosum
cca   Cortex cingularis
cd   Nucleus caudatus
csr   Colliculus superior
ep   Epiphysis
fd   Fascia dentata hippocampi
fh   Fimbria hippocampi
frp   Formatio reticularis pontis
frtm Formatio reticularis tegmenti mesencephali
gc   Substantia grisea centralis
gh   Gyrus hippocampi
gpo   Griseum pontis
hip   Hippocampus
mv   Nucleus mesencephalicus n. trigemini
na   Nucleus arcuati
nci   Nucleus colliculi inferioris
ncs   Nucleus centralis superior
nll   Nucleus lemnisci lateralis
nt   Nucleus n. trochlearis
os   Nucleus olivaris superior
pg   Nucleus parabigeminalis
pvi   Nucleus pulvinaris inferior thalami
pvl   Nucleus pulvinaris lateralis thalami
pvm   Nucleus pulvinaris medialis thalami
st   Stria terminalis

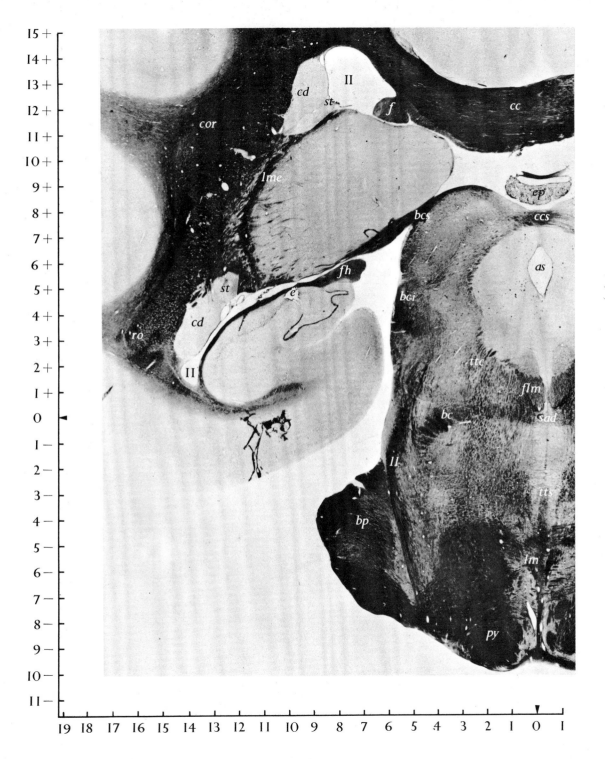

as	Aquaeductus Sylvii
bc	Brachium conjunctivum
bci	Brachium colliculi inferioris
bcs	Brachium colliculi superioris
bp	Brachium pontis
cc	Corpus callosum
ccs	Commissura colliculi superioris
cd	Nucleus caudatus
cor	Corona radiata
e	Electrode track
ep	Epiphysis
f	Fornix
fh	Fimbria hippocampi
flm	Fasciculus longitudinalis medialis
ll	Lemniscus lateralis
lm	Lemniscus medialis
lme	Lamina medullaris externa thalami
py	Tractus pyramidalis
ro	Radiatio optica
sad	Striae acusticae dorsalis
st	Stria terminalis
ttc	Tractus tegmentalis centralis
tts	Tractus tectospinalis
II	Ventriculus lateralis

67

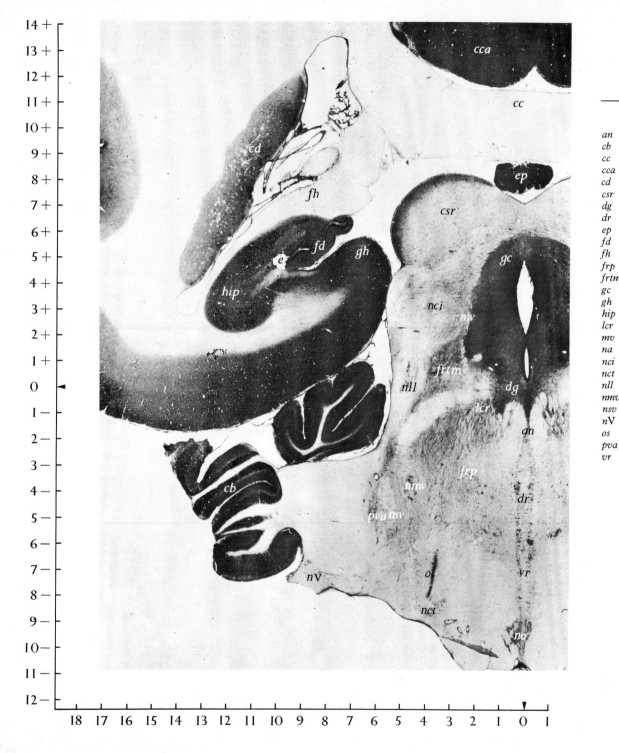

A 0·5 C

an   Nucleus annularis
cb   Cerebellum
cc   Corpus callosum
cca   Cortex cingularis
cd   Nucleus caudatus
csr   Colliculus superior
dg   Nucleus dorsalis tegmenti (Gudden)
dr   Nucleus dorsalis raphae
ep   Epiphysis
fd   Fascia dentata hippocampi
fh   Fimbria hippocampi
frp   Formatio reticularis pontis
frtm   Formatio reticularis tegmenti mesencephali
gc   Substantia grisea centralis
gh   Gyrus hippocampi
hip   Hippocampus
lcr   Locus coeruleus
mv   Nucleus mesencephalicus n. trigemini
na   Nucleus arcuati
nci   Nucleus colliculi inferioris
nct   Nucleus trapezoidalis
nll   Nucleus lemnisci lateralis
nmv   Nucleus motorius n. trigemini
nsv   Nucleus tractus spinalis n. trigemini
nV   Nervus trigeminus
os   Nucleus olivaris superior
pva   Nucleus principalis n. trigemini
vr   Nucleus ventralis raphae

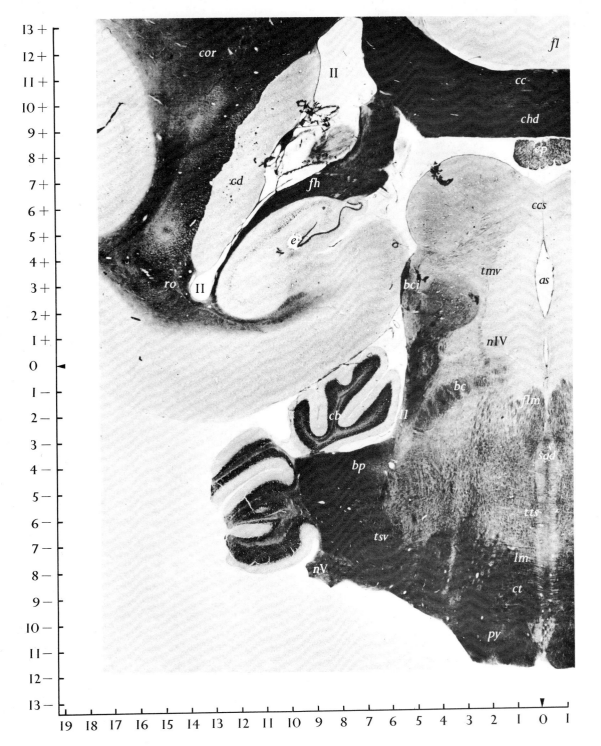

as	Aquaeductus Sylvii
bc	Brachium conjunctivum
bci	Brachium colliculi inferioris
bp	Brachium pontis
cb	Cerebellum
cc	Corpus callosum
ccs	Commissura colliculi superioris
cd	Nucleus caudatus
chd	Commissura hippocampi dorsalis
cor	Corona radiata
ct	Corpus trapezoideum
ep	Epiphysis
fh	Fimbria hippocampi
fl	Fissura longitudinalis cerebri
flm	Fasciculus longitudinalis medialis
ll	Lemniscus lateralis
lm	Lemniscus medialis
*n*IV	Nervus trochlearis
*n*V	Nervus trigeminus
py	Tractus pyramidalis
ro	Radiatio optica
sad	Striae acusticae dorsalis
tmv	Tractus mesencephalicus n. trigemini
tsv	Tractus spinalis n. trigemini
tts	Tractus tectospinalis
II	Ventriculus lateralis

AP 0·0 C

cb	Cerebellum
cc	Corpus callosum
cd	Nucleus caudatus
cds	Nucleus cochlearis dorsalis
chd	Commissura hippocampi, pars dorsalis
csr	Colliculus superior
cvs	Nucleus cochlearis ventralis
dr	Nucleus dorsalis raphae
ep	Epiphysis
fd	Fascia dentata hippocampi
fh	Fimbria hippocampi
fl	Fissura longitudinalis cerebri
flc	Flocculus cerebelli
frg	Nucleus reticularis magnocellularis
frs	Nucleus reticularis parvocellularis
gc	Substantia grisea centralis
gh	Gyrus hippocampi
hip	Hippocampus
mv	Nucleus mesencephalicus n. trigemini
nci	Nucleus colliculi inferioris
nct	Nucleus corpus trapezoidalis
nf	Nucleus facialis
nla	Nucleus lateralis anuli aquaeductus
nma	Nucleus medialis anuli aquaeductus
nmv	Nucleus motorius n. trigemini
nsv	Nucleus tractus spinalis n. trigemini
oi	Nucleus olivaris inferior
pbl	Nucleus parabrachialis lateralis
pbm	Nucleus parabrachialis medialis
pfl	Paraflocculus cerebelli
pva	Nucleus principalis n. trigemini
vr	Nucleus ventralis raphae

70

AP 0·0 W

as	Aquaeductus Sylvii
bc	Brachium conjunctivum
bci	Brachium colliculi inferioris
bp	Brachium pontis
cc	Corpus callosum
cci	Commissura colliculi inferioris
cd	Nucleus caudatus
chd	Commissura hippocampi, pars dorsalis
ep	Epiphysis
fh	Fimbria hippocampi
flm	Fasciculus longitudinalis medialis
ll	Lemniscus lateralis
lm	Lemniscus medialis
ntr	Nervus trigemini radix motoria
nIV	Nervus trochlearis
nV	Nervus trigeminus
nVII	Nervus facialis
py	Tractus pyramidalis
tmv	Tractus mesencephalicus n. trigemini
tst	Tractus spinothalamicus
tsv	Tractus spinalis n. trigemini
tts	Tractus tectospinalis
II	Ventriculus lateralis

71

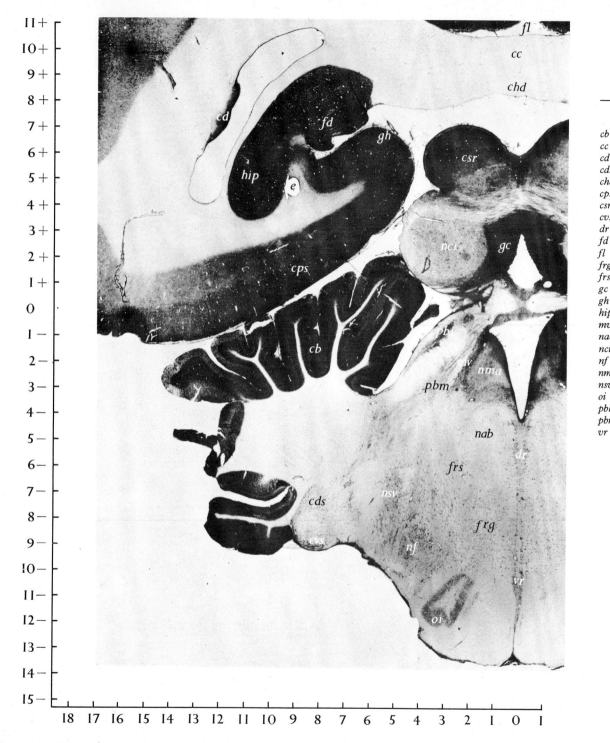

P 0·5 C

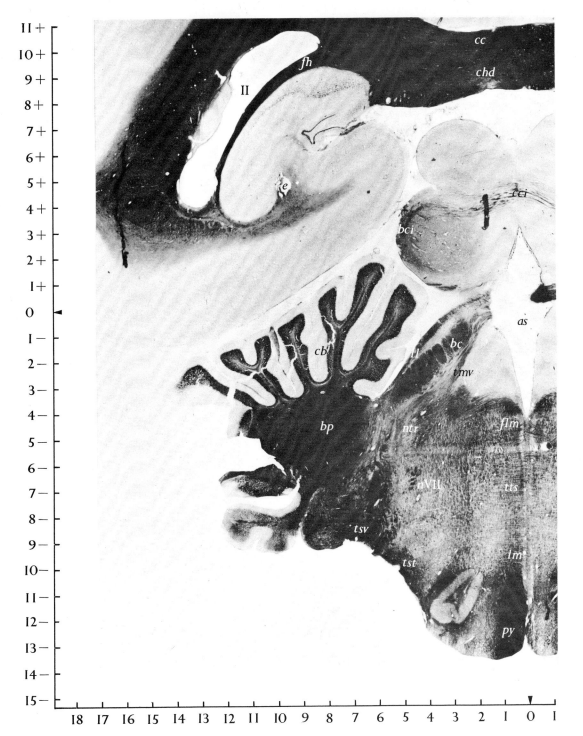

as   Aquaeductus Sylvii
bc   Brachium conjunctivum
bci   Brachium colliculi inferioris
bp   Brachium pontis
cb   Cerebellum
cc   Corpus callosum
cci   Commissura colliculi inferioris
chd   Commissura hippocampi, pars dorsalis
e   Electrode track
fh   Fimbria hippocampi
flm   Fasciculus longitudinalis medialis
ll   Lemniscus lateralis
lm   Lemniscus medialis
ntr   Nervus trigemini radix motoria
nVII   Nervus facialis
py   Tractus pyramidalis
tmv   Tractus mesencephalicus n. trigemini
tst   Tractus spinothalamicus
tsv   Tractus spinalis n. trigemini
tts   Tractus tectospinalis
II   Ventriculus lateralis

73

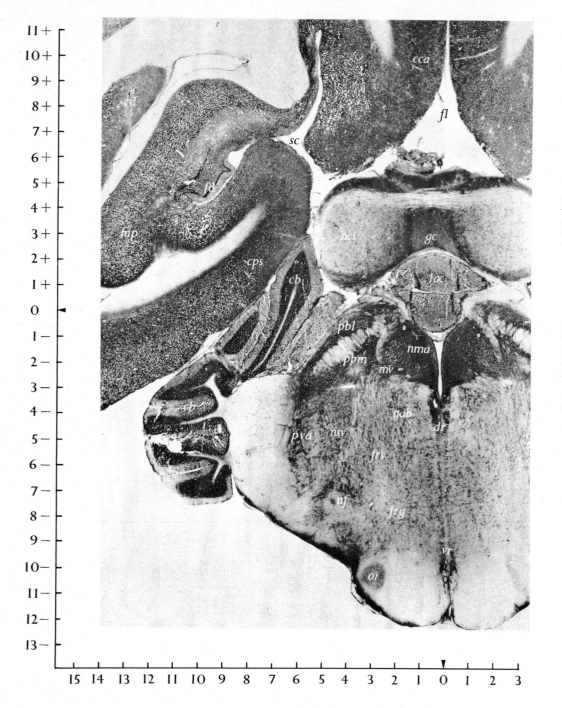

P 1·5 C

cb   Cerebellum
cca   Cortex cingularis
cd   Nucleus caudatus
cps   Cortex praestriatus
dr   Nucleus dorsalis raphae
fd   Fascia dentata
fl   Fissura longitudinalis cerebri
frg   Nucleus reticularis magnocellularis
frs   Nucleus reticularis parvocellularis
gc   Substantia grisea centralis
hip   Hippocampus
lac   Lobus anterior (cerebelli)
mv   Nucleus tractus mesencephali n. trigemini
nab   Nucleus n. abducentis
nci   Nucleus colliculi inferioris
nf   Nucleus n. facialis
nma   Nucleus medialis anuli aquaeductus
nsv   Nucleus tractus spinalis n. trigemini
oi   Nucleus olivaris inferior
pbl   Nucleus parabrachialis lateralis
pbm   Nucleus parabrachialis medialis
pva   Nucleus principalis n. trigemini
sc   Sulcus calcarinus
vr   Nucleus ventralis raphae

74

P 1·5 W

bc   Brachium conjunctivum
bci   Brachium colliculi inferioris
bp   Brachium pontis
cb   Cerebellum
cci   Commissura colliculi inferioris
crf   Corpus restiforme
fh   Fimbria hippocampi
fl   Fissura longitudinalis cerebri
flm   Fasciculus longitudinalis medialis
ll   Lemniscus lateralis
lm   Lemniscus medialis
nIV   Nervus trochlearis
nVII   Nervus facialis
nVIII   Nervus vestibularis
py   Tractus pyramidalis
scp   Tractus spinocerebellaris posterior
tmv   Tractus mesencephalicus n. trigemini
tst   Tractus spinothalamicus
tsv   Tractus spinalis n. trigemini
tts   Tractus tectospinalis
II   Ventriculus lateralis
IV   Ventriculus quartus

75

P 2·5 C

cb   Cerebellum
cd   Nucleus caudatus
cds   Nucleus cochlearis dorsalis
cir   Colliculus inferior
cps   Cortex praestriatus
dr   Nucleus dorsalis raphae
fd   Fascia dentata
fl   Fissura longitudinalis cerebri
flc   Flocculus (cerebelli)
frg   Nucleus reticularis magnocellularis
frs   Nucleus reticularis parvocellularis
hip   Hippocampus
lac   Lobus anterior (cerebelli)
nab   Nucleus n. abducentis
nf   Nucleus n. facialis
nma   Nucleus medialis anuli aquaeductus
nsv   Nucleus tractus spinalis n. trigemini
nVIIIA Nervus acusticus
oi   Nucleus olivaris inferior
oid   Nucleus olivaris inferior dorsalis
oim   Nucleus olivaris inferior medialis
pbl   Nucleus parabrachialis lateralis
pbm   Nucleus parabrachialis medialis
pfl   Paraflocculus (cerebelli)
pva   Nucleus principalis n. trigemini
sc   Sulcus calcarinus
vr   Nucleus ventralis raphae

76.

P 2·5 W

bc	Brachium conjunctivum
bp	Brachium pontis
cir	Colliculus inferior
crf	Corpus restiforme
fl	Fissura longitudinalis cerebri
flm	Fasciculus longitudinalis medialis
lac	Lobus anterior (cerebelli)
lm	Lemniscus medialis
nVIIA	Nervus facialis (genu)
nVIIIA	Nervus acusticus
py	Tractus pyramidalis
sc	Sulcus calcarinus
sca	Tractus spinocerebellaris anterior
scp	Tractus spinocerebellaris posterior
toc	Tractus olivocerebellaris
tst	Tractus spinothalamicus
tsv	Tractus spinalis n. trigemini
tts	Tractus tectospinalis
II	Ventriculus lateralis
IV	Ventriculus quartus

P 4·0 C

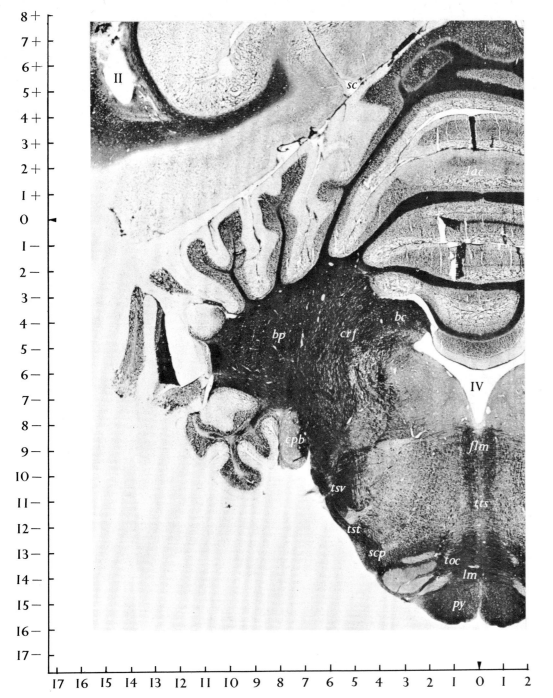

P 4·0 W

bc	Brachium conjunctivum
bp	Brachium pontis
cpb	Corpus pontobulbare
crf	Corpus restiforme
flm	Fasciculus longitudinalis medialis
lac	Lobus anterior (cerebelli)
lm	Lemniscus medialis
py	Tractus pyramidalis
sc	Sulcus calcarinus
scp	Tractus spinocerebellaris posterior
toc	Tractus olivocerebellaris
tst	Tractus spinothalamicus
tsv	Tractus spinalis n. trigemini
tts	Tractus tectospinalis
II	Ventriculus lateralis
IV	Ventriculus quartus

79

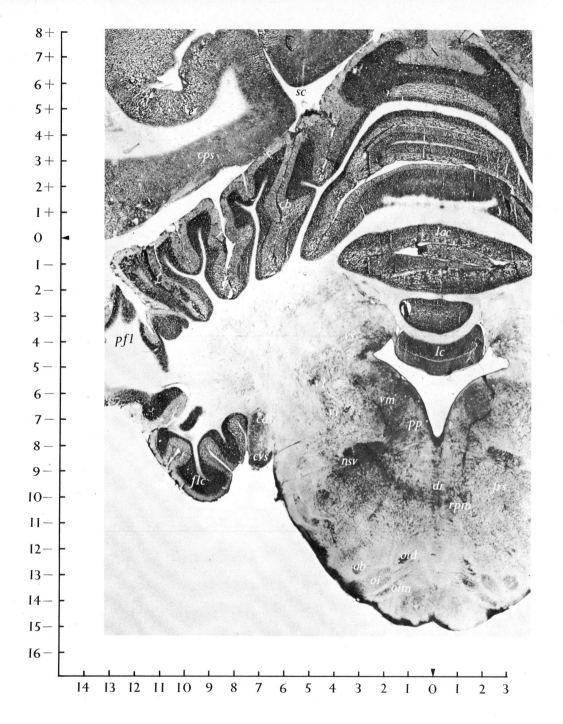

ab	Nucleus ambiguus
cb	Cerebellum
cds	Nucleus cochlearis dorsalis
cps	Cortex praestriatus
cvs	Nucleus cochlearis ventralis
dr	Nucleus dorsalis raphae
flc	Flocculus (cerebelli)
frs	Nucleus reticularis parvocellularis
lac	Lobus anterior (cerebelli)
lc	Lingula cerebelli
nsv	Nucleus tractus spinalis n. trigemini
oi	Nucleus olivaris inferior
oid	Nucleus olivaris inferior dorsalis
oim	Nucleus olivaris inferior medialis
pfl	Paraflocculus (cerebelli)
pp	Nucleus praepositus
rpm	Nucleus reticularis paramedianus myelencephali
sc	Sulcus calcarinus
vi	Nucleus vestibularis inferior
vl	Nucleus vestibularis lateralis
vm	Nucleus vestibularis medialis
vs	Nucleus vestibularis superior

P 4·5 W

bc   Brachium conjunctivum
bp   Brachium pontis
cb   Cerebellum
cpb   Corpus pontobulbare
crf   Corpus restiforme
flm   Fasciculus longitudinalis medialis
lc   Lingula cerebelli
lm   Lemniscus medialis
nVII Nervus facialis
py   Tractus pyramidalis
rdv   Radices descendentes n. vestibularis
sc   Sulcus calcarinus
scp   Tractus spinocerebellaris posterior
toc   Tractus olivocerebellaris
tst   Tractus spinothalamicus
tsv   Tractus spinalis n. trigemini
tts   Tractus tectospinalis
IV   Ventriculus quartus

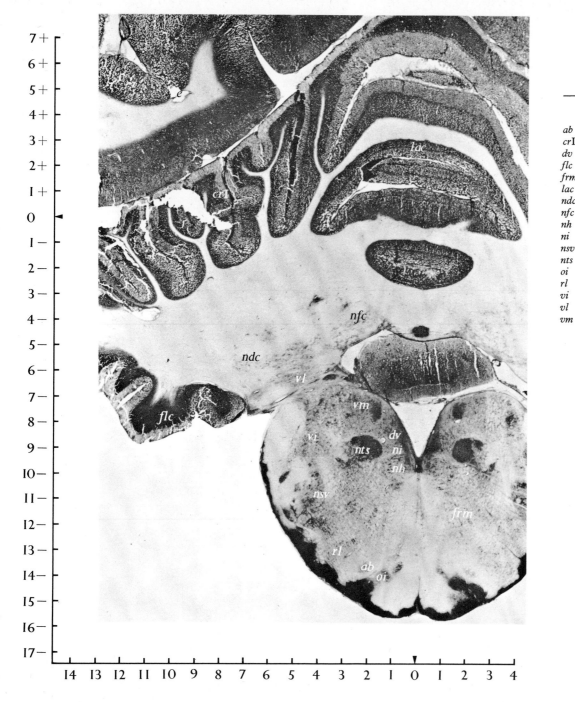

ab	Nucleus ambiguus
*cr*I	Crus I (cerebelli)
dv	Nucleus dorsalis n. vagi
flc	Flocculus (cerebelli)
frm	Formatio reticularis myelencephali
lac	Lobus anterior (cerebelli)
ndc	Nucleus dentatus cerebelli
nfc	Nucleus fastigii cerebelli
nh	Nucleus n. hypoglossi
ni	Nucleus intercalatus
nsv	Nucleus tractus spinalis n. trigemini
nts	Nucleus tractus solitarii
oi	Nucleus olivaris inferior
rl	Nucleus reticularis lateralis
vi	Nucleus vestibularis inferior
vl	Nucleus vestibularis lateralis
vm	Nucleus vestibularis medialis

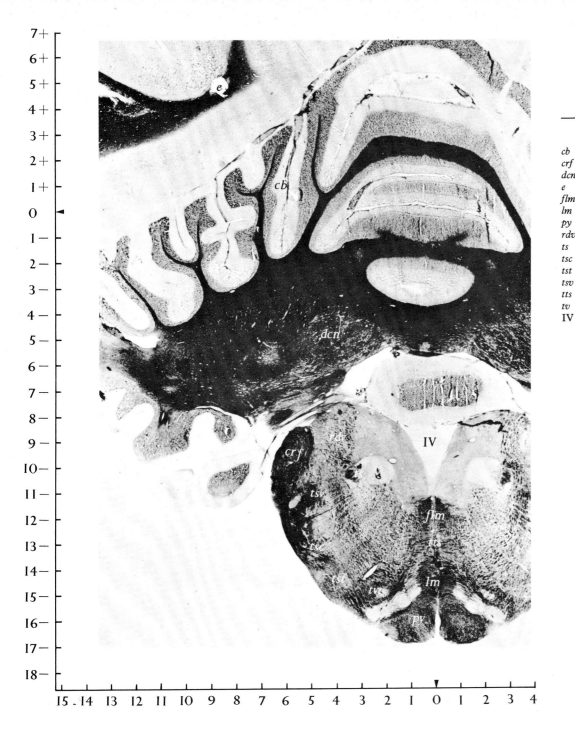

P 5·5 W

cb   Cerebellum
crf   Corpus restiforme
dcn   Deep cerebellar nuclei
e   Electrode track
flm   Fasciculus longitudinalis medialis
lm   Lemniscus medialis
py   Tractus pyramidalis
rdv   Radices descendentes n. vestibularis
ts   Tractus solitarius
tsc   Tractus spinocerebellaris
tst   Tractus spinothalamicus
tsv   Tractus spinalis n. trigemini
tts   Tractus tectospinalis
tv   Tractus vestibulospinalis
IV   Ventriculus quartus

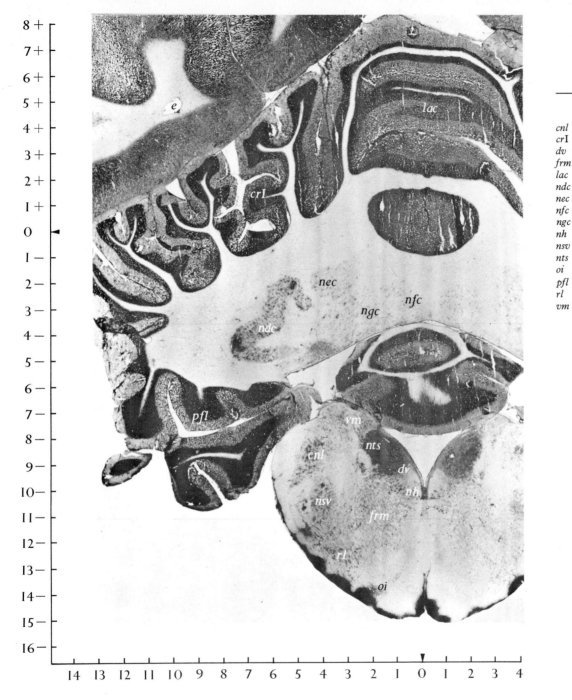

cnl   Nucleus cuneatus lateralis
crI   Crus I (cerebelli)
dv   Nucleus dorsalis n. vagi
frm   Formatio reticularis myelencephali
lac   Lobus anterior (cerebelli)
ndc   Nucleus dentatus cerebelli
nec   Nucleus emboliformis cerebelli
nfc   Nucleus fastigii cerebelli
ngc   Nucleus globosus cerebelli
nh   Nucleus n. hypoglossi
nsv   Nucleus tractus spinalis n. trigemini
nts   Nucleus tractus solitarii
oi   Nucleus olivaris inferior
pfl   Paraflocculus cerebelli
rl   Nucleus reticularis lateralis
vm   Nucleus vestibularis medialis

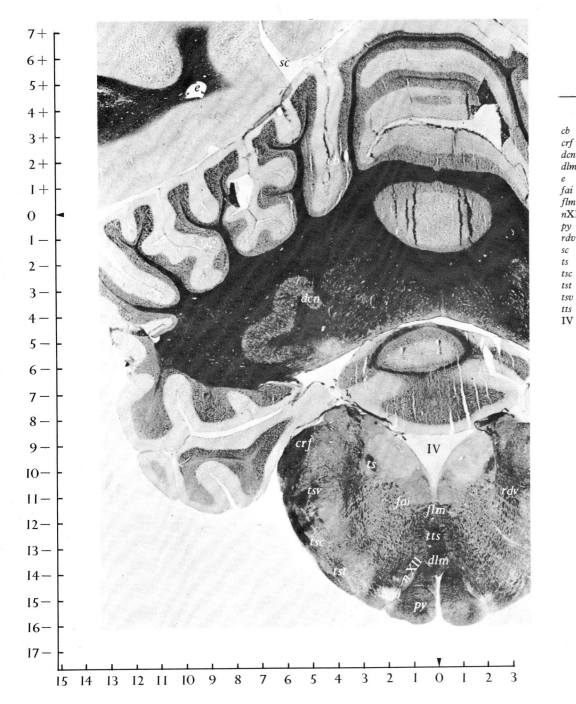

cb	Cerebellum
crf	Corpus restiforme
dcn	Deep cerebellar nuclei
dlm	Decussatio lemnisci medialis
e	Electrode track
fai	Fibrae arcuatae internae
flm	Fasciculus longitudinalis medialis
nXII	Nervus hypoglossus
py	Tractus pyramidalis
rdv	Radices descendentes n. vestibularis
sc	Sulcus calcarinus
ts	Tractus solitarius
tsc	Tractus spinocerebellaris
tst	Tractus spinothalamicus
tsv	Tractus spinalis n. trigemini
tts	Tractus tectospinalis
IV	Ventriculus quartus

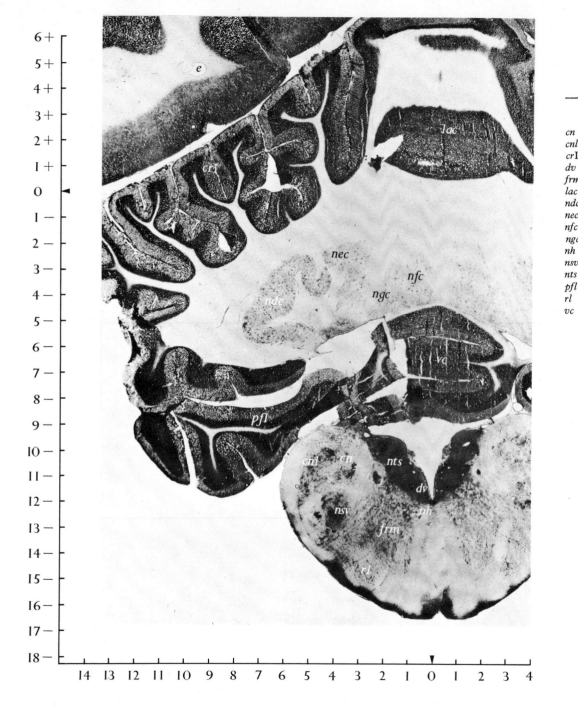

P 7·0 C

cn — Nucleus cuneatus
cnl — Nucleus cuneatus lateralis
crI — Crus I (cerebelli)
dv — Nucleus dorsalis n. vagi
frm — Formatio reticularis myelencephali
lac — Lobus anterior (cerebelli)
ndc — Nucleus dentatus cerebelli
nec — Nucleus emboliformis cerebelli
nfc — Nucleus fastigii cerebelli
ngc — Nucleus globosus cerebelli
nh — Nucleus n. hypoglossi
nsv — Nucleus tractus spinalis n. trigemini
nts — Nucleus tractus solitarii
pfl — Paraflocculus cerebelli
rl — Nucleus reticularis lateralis
vc — Vermis cerebelli

86

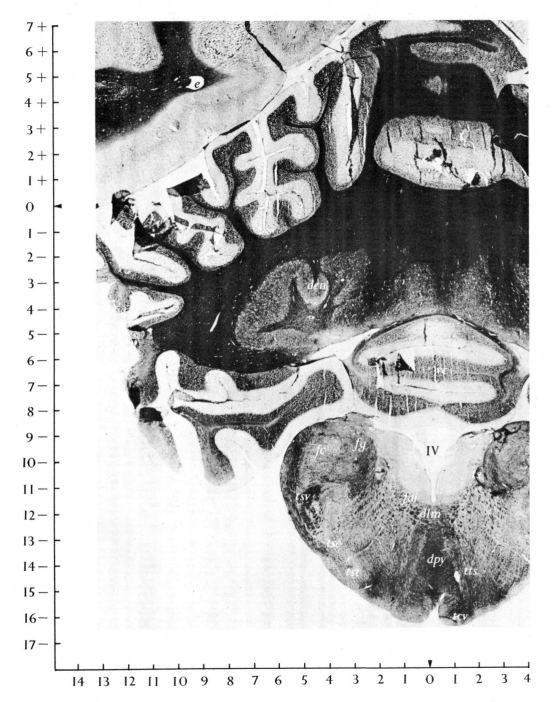

dcn Deep cerebellar nuclei
dlm Decussatio lemnisci medialis
dpy Decussatio pyramidum
e   Electrode track
fai Fibrae arcuatae internae
fc   Funiculus cuneatus
fg   Funiculus gracilis
tcv Tractus corticospinalis ventralis
ts   Tractus solitarius
tsc Tractus spinocerebellaris
tst Tractus spinothalamicus
tsv Tractus spinalis n. trigemini
tts Tractus tectospinalis
vc   Vermis cerebelli
IV   Ventriculus quartus

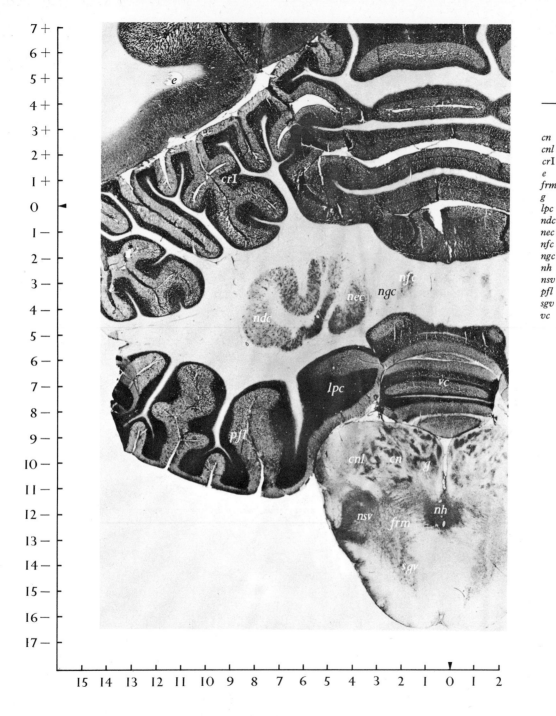

cn	Nucleus cuneatus
cnl	Nucleus cuneatus lateralis
*cr*I	Crus I (cerebelli)
e	Electrode track
frm	Formatio reticularis myelencephali
g	Nucleus gracilis
lpc	Lobus paramedianus cerebelli
ndc	Nucleus dentatus cerebelli
nec	Nucleus emboliformis cerebelli
nfc	Nucleus fastigii cerebelli
ngc	Nucleus globosus cerebelli
nh	Nucleus n. hypoglossi
nsv	Nucleus tractus spinalis n. trigemini
pfl	Paraflocculus cerebelli
sgv	Nucleus substantiae griseae ventralis
vc	Vermis cerebelli

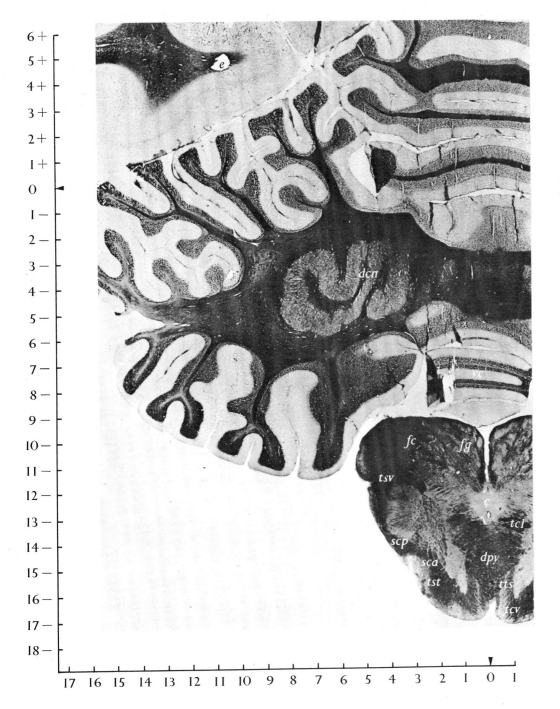

c	Canalis centralis
dcn	Deep cerebellar nuclei
dpy	Decussatio pyramidum
e	Electrode track
fc	Funiculus cuneatus
fg	Funiculus gracilis
sca	Tractus spinocerebellaris anterior
scp	Tractus spinocerebellaris posterior
tcl	Tractus corticospinalis lateralis
tcv	Tractus corticospinalis ventralis
tst	Tractus spinothalamicus
tsv	Tractus spinalis n. trigemini
tts	Tractus tectospinalis
vc	Vermis cerebelli

Key to Plates and Stereotaxic Levels

Abbreviation	Explanation	Stereotaxic levels
aaa	Area anterior amygdalae	A19·5–A15·5
ab	Nucleus ambiguus	P4·0–P5·5
aca	Area claustralis amygdalae	A19·5
ad	Nucleus anterior dorsalis thalami	A12·5–A7·5
adh	Area dorsalis hypothalami	A14·5–A10·5
ah	Nucleus anterior hypothalami	A15·5
al	Ansa lenticularis	A14·5–A11·5
alh	Area lateralis hypothalami	A15·5–A10·5
am	Nucleus anterior medialis thalami	A12·0–A10·5
amh	Area medialis hypothalami	A15·5–A14·0
an	Nucleus annularis	A6·5–A0·5
ao	Area olfactoria	A19·5–A17·0
aph	Area posterior hypothalami	A9·5
apl	Area praeoptica lateralis	A16·5
apm	Area praeoptica medialis	A16·5
apt	Area praetectalis	A4·5–A3·5
as	Aquaeductus Sylvii	A4·5–P0·5
ase	Area septalis	A19·5–A15·5
ast	Nucleus accumbens septi	A17·0–A16·5
at	Area tegmentalis	A13·0–A6·0
av	Nucleus anterior ventralis thalami	A12·5–A10·5
ba	Nucleus basalis amygdalae	A19·5–A12·5
baa	Nucleus basalis accessorius amygdalae	A19·5–A13·0
bal	Nucleus basalis accessorius lateralis amygdalae	A17·0–A14·5
bam	Nucleus basalis accessorius medialis amygdalae	A17·0–A14·5
bc	Brachium conjunctivum	A6·5–P4·5
bci	Brachium colliculi inferioris	A4·5–P1·5
bcs	Brachium colliculi superioris	A4·5–A2·0
bla	Nucleus basalis lateralis amygdalae	A17·0–A14·5
bm	Nucleus basalis (Meynert)	A17·0–A13·0
bma	Nucleus basalis medialis amygdalae	A17·0–A14·5
bp	Brachium pontis	A7·0–P4·5
c	Canalis centralis	P9·0
ca	Commissura anterior	A17·0–A14·5
cag	Nucleus corticalis amygdalae	A19·5–A13·0
cam	Corpus amygdalae	A19·5–A12·5
cb	Cerebellum	A0·5–P6·5
cc	Corpus callosum	A19·5–P0·5
cca	Cortex cingularis anterior	A17·0–P1·5
ccg	Cingulum	A11·5–A10·5
cci	Commissura colliculi inferioris	AP0·0–P1·5
ccs	Commissura colliculi superioris	A2·0–A0·5
cd	Nucleus caudatus	A19·5–P2·5
cds	Nucleus cochlearis dorsalis	AP0·0–P4·5
ce	Capsula externa	A19·5–A5·5

Abbreviation	Explanation	Stereotaxic levels
cea	Nucleus centralis amygdalae	A19·5–A14·5
cei	Nucleus centralis inferior thalami	A11·5–A6·0
cel	Nucleus centralis lateralis thalami	A8·0–A5·5
cem	Nucleus centralis medialis thalami	A11·5–A8·5
cet	Capsula extrema	A19·5–A9·5
cf	Columna fornicis	A16·5–A14·0
ch	Commissura habenulae	A3·5–A2·5
chd	Commissura hippocampi dorsalis	A0·5–P0·5
cho	Chiasma nervorum opticorum	A19·5–A15·5
ci	Capsula interna	A19·5–A5·5
cii	Nucleus centralis intermedius thalami	A11·5–A9·5
cir	Colliculus inferior	P2·5
cis	Cortex insularis	A19·5–A10·5
cl	Claustrum	A19·5–A10·5
cm	Centrum medianum thalami	A8·5–A5·5
cmm	Corpus mamillare	A11·0–A10·5
cn	Nucleus cuneatus	P7·0–P9·0
cnl	Nucleus cuneatus lateralis	P6·5–P9·0
cor	Corona radiata	A19·5–A0·5
cp	Commissura posterior	A6·5–A2·5
cpb	Corpus pontobulbare	P4·0–P4·5
cpf	Cortex piriformis	A15·5–A6·5
cpl	Plexus choroidae ventriculi lateralis	A13·0–A12·5
cps	Cortex praestriatus	P0·5–P4·5
crf	Corpus restiforme	P1·5–P6·5
crI	Crus I (cerebelli)	P5·5–P9·0
cs	Nucleus centralis superior thalami	A12·5–A5·5
csd	Commissura supraoptica dorsalis	A14·5–A12·5
csl	Nucleus centralis superior lateralis thalami	A9·5–A6·0
csm	Commissura supramamillaris	A9·5
csr	Colliculus superior	A3·0–P0·5
ct	Corpus trapezoideum	A0·5
ctp	Cortex temporalis	A19·5–A10·5
cvs	Nucleus cochlearis ventralis	AP0·0–P4·5
dbc	Decussatio brachii conjunctivi	A6·5–A2·5
dcn	Deep cerebellar nuclei	P5·5–P9·0
ddt	Decussatio dorsalis tegmenti	A6·0–A4·5
ddv	Decussatio ventralis tegmenti	A7·0
dg	Nucleus dorsalis tegmenti (Gudden)	A0·5
dlm	Decussatio lemnisci medialis	P6·5–P7·0
dmh	Nucleus dorsalis medialis hypothalami	A13·0–A12·0
dpy	Decussatio pyramidum	P7·0–P9·0
dr	Nucleus dorsalis raphae	A0·5–P4·5
ds	Nucleus dorsalis septi	A19·5–A15·5
dv	Nucleus dorsalis n. vagi	P5·5–P7·0

Abbreviation	Explanation	Stereotaxic levels
em	Eminentia medialis	A14·0–A12·0
ep	Epiphysis	A2·0–AP0·0
f	Fornix	A14·5–A2·0
fai	Fibrae arcuatae internae	P6·5–P7·0
fc	Funiculus cuneatus	P7·0–P9·0
fd	Fascia dentata hippocampi	A11·5–P2·5
fdb	Fasciculus diagonalis Broca	A19·5–A17·0
fg	Funiculus gracilis	P7·0–P9·0
fh	Fimbria hippocampi	A12·5–P1·5
fl	Fissura longitudinalis cerebri	A19·5–P2·5
flc	Flocculus (cerebelli)	AP0·0–P5·5
flm	Fasciculus longitudinalis medialis	A6·5–P6·5
fmp	Fasciculus mamillaris princeps	A10·5
frg	Nucleus reticularis magnocellularis	AP0·0–P4·0
frm	Formatio reticularis myelencephali	P5·5–P9·0
frp	Formatio reticularis pontis	A3·5–A0·5
frs	Nucleus reticularis parvocellularis	AP0·0–P4·5
frtm	Formatio reticularis tegmenti mesencephali	A8·0–A0·5
fs	Fissura lateralis cerebri (Sylvii)	A7·5–A5·5
ftp	Fibrae pontis transversae	A7·0–A2·5
fu	Fasciculus uncinatus	A19·5–A16·5
g	Nucleus gracilis	P9·0
gc	Substantia grisea centralis	A4·5–P1·5
gh	Gyrus hippocampi	A13·0–P0·5
gl	Corpus geniculatum laterale	A9·5–A5·5
glo	Corpus geniculatum laterale, pars oralis	A7·5
gm	Corpus geniculatum mediale	A7·5–A3·0
gmm	Corpus geniculatum mediale, pars magnocellularis	A4·5
gp	Globus pallidus	A17·0–A9·5
gph	Griseum periventriculare hypothalami	A12·5–A9·5
gpm	Griseum periventriculare mesencephali	A8·5–A5·5
gpo	Griseum pontis	A6·5–A2·0
gu	Gyrus uncinatus	A19·5–A8·5
h	Campus Foreli	A11·5–A7·5
h₁	Campus Foreli, pars dorsalis	A12·0–A7·5
h₂	Campus Foreli, pars ventralis	A12·0–A7·5
hip	Hippocampus	A13·0–P2·5
hl	Nucleus habenularis lateralis epithalami	A4·5–A3·5
hm	Nucleus habenularis medialis epithalami	A4·5–A2·5
ic	Insula Callejae	A19·5
ica	Nucleus intercalatus amygdalae	A14·5–A14·0
ih	Nucleus infundibularis hypothalami	A14·0–A12·5
ip	Nucleus interpeduncularis	A8·5–A3·0
is	Nucleus interstitialis (Cajal)	A7·5–A7·0
la	Nucleus lateralis amygdalae	A19·5–A12·5

Abbreviation	Explanation	Stereotaxic levels
lac	Lobus anterior (cerebelli)	P1·5–P7·0
lc	Lingula cerebelli	P4·0–P4·5
lcr	Locus coeruleus	A0·5
ld	Nucleus lateralis dorsalis thalami	A9·5–A5·5
lge	Globus pallidus, lamina medullaris externa	A17·0–A8·5
lgi	Globus pallidus, lamina medullaris interna	A14·5–A11·5
ll	Lemniscus lateralis	A2·5–P1·5
lm	Lemniscus medialis	A7·0–P5·5
lme	Lamina medullaris externa thalami	A13·0–A2·0
lmi	Lamina medullaris interna thalami	A12·5–A5·5
lmt	Nucleus limitans thalami	A4·5–A3·0
lp	Nucleus lateralis posterior thalami	A8·0–A5·5
lpc	Lobus paramedianus cerebelli	P9·0
ls	Nucleus lateralis septi	A19·5–A15·5
ma	Nucleus medialis amygdalae	A19·5–A12·0
md	Nucleus medialis dorsalis thalami	A12·5–A3·5
mi	Nucleus intermedius corpus mamillaris	A11·5–A10·5
ml	Nucleus lateralis corpus mamillaris	A11·5–A10·5
mm	Nucleus medialis corpus mamillaris	A11·5–A10·5
ms	Nucleus medialis septi	A19·5–A15·5
mv	Nucleus tractus mesencephali n. trigemini	A2·5–P1·5
na	Nucleus arcuati	A2·0–A0·5
nab	Nucleus n. abducentis	P0·5–P2·5
nca	Nucleus commissurae anterioris	A17·0–A15·5
nci	Nucleus colliculi inferioris	A2·5–P1·5
ncs	Nucleus centralis superior	A2·5–A2·0
nct	Nucleus trapezoidalis	A0·5–AP0·0
ndc	Nucleus dentatus cerebelli	P5·5–P9·0
ndk	Nucleus Darkschewitsch	A8·0
nec	Nucleus emboliformis cerebelli	P6·5–P9·0
nf	Nucleus n. facialis	AP0·0–P2·5
nfc	Nucleus fastigii cerebelli	P5·5–P9·0
nfdb	Nucleus fasciculi diagonalis Broca	A19·5–A15·5
ngc	Nucleus globosus cerebelli	P6·5–P9·0
nh	Nucleus n. hypoglossi	P5·5–P9·0
ni	Nucleus intercalatus	P5·5
nla	Nucleus lateralis anuli aquaeductus	AP0·0
nll	Nucleus lemnisci lateralis	A3·0–A0·5
nma	Nucleus medialis anuli aquaeductus	AP0·0–P2·5
nmv	Nucleus motorius n. trigemini	A0·5–AP0·0
noc	Nucleus centralis n. oculomotorii	A7·5–A3·5
nod	Nucleus n. oculomotorii, pars dorsalis	A7·5–A3·5
nov	Nucleus n. oculomotorii, pars ventralis	A7·5–A3·5
now	Nucleus rostralis n. oculomotorii (Westphal–Edinger)	A8·0
nr	Nucleus ruber	A8·5–A5·5

Abbreviation	Explanation	Stereotaxic levels
nst	Nucleus striae terminalis	A15·5–A12·5
nsth	Nucleus subthalamicus	A10·5–A8·0
nstt	Nucleus supratrochlearis	A3·0–A2·5
nsv	Nucleus tractus spinalis n. trigemini	A0·5–P9·0
nt	Nucleus n. trochlearis	A3·0–A2·0
ntr	Nervus n. trigemini radix motoria	AP0·0–P0·5
nts	Nucleus tractus solitarii	P5·5–P7·0
*n*III	Nervus oculomotorius	A8·5–A7·5
*n*IV	Nervus trochlearis	A0·5–P1·5
*n*V	Nervus trigeminus	A0·5–AP0·0
*n*VII	Nervus facialis	AP0·0–P4·5
*n*VIIA	Nervus facialis (genu)	P2·5
*n*VIII	Nervus vestibularis	P1·5
*n*VIIIA	Nervus acusticus	P2·5
*n*XII	Nervus hypoglossus	P6·5
oi	Nucleus olivaris inferior	AP0·0–P6·5
oid	Nucleus olivaris inferior dorsalis	P2·5–P4·5
oim	Nucleus olivaris inferior medialis	P2·5–P4·5
os	Nucleus olivaris superior	A2·0–A0·5
pbl	Nucleus parabrachialis lateralis	AP0·0–P2·5
pbm	Nucleus parabrachialis medialis	AP0·0–P2·5
pc	Nucleus paracentralis thalami	A9·5–A8·5
pcm	Pedunculus corporis mamillaris	A10·5
pcr	Pedunculus cerebri	A11·5–A6·0
pd	Nucleus peripeduncularis thalami	A7·5–A6·5
pf	Nucleus parafascicularis thalami	A8·0–A6·0
pfl	Paraflocculus (cerebelli)	AP0·0–P9·0
pg	Nucleus parabigeminalis	A3·0–A2·0
ph	Nucleus paraventricularis hypothalami	A14·5–A13·0
pm	Nucleus praeopticus medianus	A17·0–A15·5
po	Pons	A7·0–A5·5
pp	Nucleus praepositus	P4·0–P4·5
pt	Nucleus parataenialis thalami	A12·5–A9·5
pti	Pedunculus thalami inferior	A13·0–A12·5
put	Putamen	A19·5–A4·5
pv	Nucleus paraventricularis thalami	A12·0–A5·5
pva	Nucleus principalis n. trigemini	A0·5–P2·5
pvi	Nucleus pulvinaris inferior thalami	A4·5–A2·0
pvl	Nucleus pulvinaris lateralis thalami	A4·5–A2·0
pvm	Nucleus pulvinaris medialis thalami	A4·5–A2·0
pvo	Nucleus pulvinaris oralis thalami	A6·5–A5·5
py	Tractus pyramidalis	A7·0–P6·5
r	Nucleus reticularis thalami	A13·0–A2·5
ra	Radiatio acustica	A4·5–A3·0
rdv	Radices descendentes n. vestibularis	P4·5–P6·5

Abbreviation	Explanation	Stereotaxic levels
rgc	Radiatio geniculo-calcarina	A10·5–A5·5
rgt	Radiatio geniculo-temporalis	A4·5
rl	Nucleus reticularis lateralis	P5·5–P7·0
ro	Radiatio optica	A7·5–A0·5
rpm	Nucleus reticularis paramedianus myelencephali	P4·5
rtp	Nucleus reticularis tegmenti pontis	A6·5–A3·0
ru	Nucleus reuniens thalami	A12·0–A10·5
sad	Striae acusticae dorsalis	A2·0–A0·5
sbc	Subiculum	A11·5–A8·5
sc	Sulcus calcarinus	P1·5–P6·5
sca	Tractus spinocerebellaris anterior	P2·5–P9·0
scp	Tractus spinocerebellaris posterior	P1·5–P9·0
sfo	Organum subfornicale	A14·5
sgv	Nucleus substantiae griseae ventralis	P9·0
sh	Nucleus suprachiasmaticus hypothalami	A15·5
si	Substantia innominata	A19·5–A11·0
sm	Stria medullaris thalami	A13·0–A4·5
smh	Nucleus supramamillaris hypothalami	A10·5
smt	Nucleus submedius thalami	A11·5–A8·0
sn	Substantia nigra	A8·0–A6·0
snc	Substantia nigra, pars compacta	A9·5–A8·5
snd	Substantia nigra, pars diffusa	A9·5–A8·5
soh	Nucleus supraopticus hypothalami	A15·5–A14·0
sol	Stria olfactoria lateralis	A19·5
som	Stria olfactoria medialis	A19·5
spa	Substantia perforata anterior	A19·5
st	Stria terminalis	A13·0–A2·0
tce	Tuber cinereum	A14·0
tcl	Tractus corticospinalis lateralis	P9·0
tcv	Tractus corticospinalis ventralis	P7·0–P9·0
tdt	Tractus dentatothalamicus	A7·0
tht	Tractus hypothalamicotegmentalis	A9·5–A7·5
tmt	Tractus mamillothalamicus	A11·0–A10·5
tmv	Tractus mesencephalicus n. trigemini	A0·5–P1·5
to	Tractus opticus	A14·5–A9·5
toc	Tractus olivocerebellaris	P2·5–P4·5
tof	Tuberculum olfactorium	A19·5–A16·5
tom	Tractus olfactomesencephalicus	A17·0–A15·5
trm	Tractus retroflexus (Meynert) (Tractus hebenulointerpeduncularis)	A7·5–A4·5
trs	Nucleus triangularis septi	A14·0–A13·0
ts	Tractus solitarius	P5·5–P7·0
tsc	Tractus spinocerebellaris	P5·5–P7·0
tst	Tractus spinothalamicus	AP0·0–P9·0
tsv	Tractus spinalis n. trigemini	A0·5–P9·0

Abbreviation	Explanation	Stereotaxic levels
ttc	Tractus tegmentalis centralis	A6·5–A2·0
ttp	Tractus tectopontinus	A4·5–A3·0
tts	Tractus tectospinalis	A2·0–P9·0
tv	Tractus vestibulospinalis	P5·5
va	Nucleus ventralis anterior thalami	A13·0–A10·5
vc	Vermis (cerebelli)	P7·0–P9·0
vi	Nucleus vestibularis inferior	P4·0–P5·5
vl	Nucleus vestibularis lateralis	P4·0–P5·5
vla	Nucleus ventralis lateralis thalami	A9·5–A8·0
vlm	Nucleus ventralis lateralis thalami, pars medialis	A9·5
vlo	Nucleus ventralis lateralis thalami, pars oralis	A11·5–A8·5
vm	Nucleus vestibularis medialis	P4·5–P6·5
vmh	Nucleus ventralis medialis hypothalami	A13·0–A12·0
vpi	Nucleus ventralis posterior inferior thalami	A8·5–A6·5
vpl	Nucleus ventralis posterior lateralis thalami	A8·5–A6·0
vpm	Nucleus ventralis posterior medialis thalami	A8·5–A6·0
vr	Nucleus ventralis raphae	A0·5–P2·5
vs	Nucleus vestibularis superior	P4·0–P4·5
zi	Zona incerta	A12·5–A8·0
II	Ventriculus lateralis	A19·5–P4·0
III	Ventriculus tertius	A16·5–A2·5
IV	Ventriculus quartus	P0·5–P7·0

PRINTED IN GREAT BRITAIN
AT THE UNIVERSITY PRESS, OXFORD
BY VIVIAN RIDLER
PRINTER TO THE UNIVERSITY